Health Effects and Exposure Assessment to Bioaerosols in Indoor and Outdoor Environments

Health Effects and Exposure Assessment to Bioaerosols in Indoor and Outdoor Environments

Editor

Ewa Bragoszewska

MDPI • Basel • Beijing • Wuhan • Barcelona • Belgrade • Manchester • Tokyo • Cluj • Tianjin

Editor
Ewa Bragoszewska
Department of Technologies and
Installations for Waste
Management
Silesian University of
Technology
Gliwice
Poland

Editorial Office
MDPI
St. Alban-Anlage 66
4052 Basel, Switzerland

This is a reprint of articles from the Special Issue published online in the open access journal *Atmosphere* (ISSN 2073-4433) (available at: www.mdpi.com/journal/atmosphere/special_issues/exposure_bioaerosol).

For citation purposes, cite each article independently as indicated on the article page online and as indicated below:

LastName, A.A.; LastName, B.B.; LastName, C.C. Article Title. *Journal Name* **Year**, *Volume Number*, Page Range.

ISBN 978-3-0365-2264-7 (Hbk)
ISBN 978-3-0365-2263-0 (PDF)

Contents

Ewa Bragoszewska
Health Effects and Exposure Assessment to Bioaerosols in Indoor and Outdoor Environments
Reprinted from: *Atmosphere* **2021**, *12*, 359, doi:10.3390/atmos12030359 . . . . **1**

Ewa Bragoszewska, Magdalena Bogacka and Krzysztof Pikoń
Effectiveness and Eco-Costs of Air Cleaners in Terms of Improving Fungal Air Pollution in Dwellings Located in Southern Poland—A Preliminary Study
Reprinted from: *Atmosphere* **2020**, *11*, 1255, doi:10.3390/atmos11111255 . . . . **3**

Marta Małecka-Adamowicz, Beata Koim-Puchowska and Ewa A. Dembowska
Diversity of Bioaerosols in Selected Rooms of Two Schools and Antibiotic Resistance of Isolated Staphylococcal Strains (Bydgoszcz, Poland): A Case Study
Reprinted from: *Atmosphere* **2020**, *11*, 1105, doi:10.3390/atmos11101105 . . . . **15**

Ewa Bragoszewska, Izabela Biedroń and Anna Mainka
Microbiological Air Quality in a Highschool Gym Located in an Urban Area of Southern Poland—Preliminary Research
Reprinted from: *Atmosphere* **2020**, *11*, 797, doi:10.3390/atmos11080797 . . . . **31**

Ewa Zender-Świercz
Microclimate in Rooms Equipped with Decentralized Façade Ventilation Device
Reprinted from: *Atmosphere* **2020**, *11*, 800, doi:10.3390/atmos11080800 . . . . **45**

Krzysztof Skowron, Katarzyna Grudlewska-Buda, Sylwia Kożuszko, Natalia Wiktorczyk, Karolina Jadwiga Skowron, Agnieszka Mikucka, Zuzanna Bernaciak and Eugenia Gospodarek-Komkowska
Efficacy of Radiant Catalytic Ionization in Reduction of *Enterococcus* spp., *Clostridioides difficile* and *Staphylococcus aureus* in Indoor Air
Reprinted from: *Atmosphere* **2020**, *11*, 764, doi:10.3390/atmos11070764 . . . . **67**

atmosphere

MDPI

ditorial

Iealth Effects and Exposure Assessment to Bioaerosols in ndoor and Outdoor Environments

wa Brągoszewska

Department of Technologies and Installations for Waste Management, Faculty of Energy and Environmental Engineering, Silesian University of Technology, 18 Konarskiego St., 44-100 Gliwice, Poland; ewa.bragoszewska@polsl.pl

The *Atmosphere* Special Issue entitled "Health Effects and Exposure Assessment to Bioaerosols in Indoor and Outdoor Environments" comprises five original papers.

Air pollution, due to natural and anthropogenic sources, generates an enormous environmental cost. The issue of healthy living spaces and good air quality is a global concern, because individuals inhale 15,000 L of air every 24 h. Thus, contemporary monitoring and reducing exposure to air pollutants presents a particular challenge for us. One of the crucial indicators of indoor and outdoor air quality is bioaerosols. They play an instrumental role as risk factors when it comes to adverse health outcome. These indicators, also known as primary biological airborne particles (PBAPs), have been linked to various health effects such as infectious diseases, toxic effects, allergies, and even cancer. PBAPs include all particles with a biological source in suspension in the air (bacteria, fungi, viruses, pollen), as well as biomolecules (toxins, debris from membranes). To foster our current scientific knowledge about bioaerosols, scientific research studies related to the characteristics of biological aerosols in indoor and outdoor environments, the methods used to improve air quality, as well as the health effects of and exposure assessment to bioaerosols problem, have been collected in this Special Issue.

itation: Brągoszewska, E. Health fects and Exposure Assessment to oaerosols in Indoor and Outdoor wironments. *Atmosphere* **2021**, *12*, 9. https://doi.org/10.3390/ mos12030359

eceived: 5 March 2021
ccepted: 8 March 2021
ıblished: 9 March 2021

The first paper in this Special Issue applied the monitoring of PBAPs collected in a high school gymnastic hall located in an urban area of Poland. Brągoszewska et al. [1] indicated that the concentrations of bacterial aerosol in the analysed high school gym in the naturally ventilated historic building were not particularly hazardous for the occupants; however, the share of the respirable fraction (particles with an aerodynamic diameter less than 3.3 μm) increased during sports activities from 30% (before gymnastic classes) to 80% of the total concentration of bacterial aerosol during physical activities. The highest antibiotic resistance was revealed to be *Staphylococcus epidermis* (isolated during gymnastic classes) and *Pseudomonas* sp. (isolated before gymnastic classes). The results of this study may indicate the usefulness of periodic PBAPs monitoring to verify the quality of the air and to establish possible technologically achievable guide levels of contamination for educational buildings. Małecka-Adamowicz et al. [2] presented a study about evaluating PBAPs in libraries, cafeterias, and selected classrooms of two schools in northern Poland and determined the antibiotic resistance of Staphylococcal strains isolated from the indoor air. A statistically significant relationship between the size of the rooms and the concentration of heterotrophic bacteria was observed. In both schools, higher microbial concentrations were recorded in smaller rooms (the cafeterias). The antibiograms indicated that resistance to erythromycin was common in 62.5% of the isolated staphylococcal strains. Levofloxacin and gentamicin were the most effective antibiotics. Given the current lack of precise indoor air quality guidelines in Poland, the research may be a very valuable contribution. Zender-Świercz [3] focused on analysing internal air parameters in an office room equipped with a decentralized façade ventilation device. The analyses of both temperature and humidity have proven that the values of inside air temperature and humidity are not affected by the temperature and humidity of outside air. In this case, the negative pressure generated during the exhaust cycle must induce an inflow of warm and dry air from an adjacent room Skowron et al. [4] presented an assessment of the efficiency of radiant catalytic ionization (RCI) in eliminating enterococci resistant to selected antibiotics in the air compared to the antibiotic-susceptible strain, antibiotic-resistant, toxinogenic *Clostridioides difficile* in comparison with the non-toxinogenic, antibiotic-susceptible strain and elimination of *Staphylococcus aureus* non-MRSA and MRSA strain. The obtained results indicate that the use of RCI may contribute to reducing the occurrence of dangerous pathogens (including MRSA) in the indoor air, and perhaps transmission and persistence in the environment, thus, it is worth noticing that the RCI device should be taken into account in the designing of ventilation systems. Brągoszewska et al. [5] introduced methods to improve indoor air quality using air purifiers with high-efficiency particulate air filters (HEPA) that remove PBAPs from indoor environments. The reduction in total concentration of fungal aerosol in the presented study even when air purifiers were active was at a level of 42%. The current findings suggested the need for further work, particularly focused on a re-emission process generated by air blown from air purifiers. The elucidation of this relationship will be an important foundation from which to develop air cleaning technologies. Moreover, this study shows the need for implementing a strategy to control and improve PBAP air quality in indoor environments.

The goal of this Special Issue was to present research with a wide perspective, involving air quality research studies, and the five papers in this Special Issue achieve. I hope that the results presented in this Special Issue will spur investigations in this area for more invigorating research in the future.

Funding: This research received no external funding.

Acknowledgments: The editor would like to thank the authors for their contributions, the reviewers for their helpful comments, and the Editorial Office for the support in publishing this Special Issue.

Conflicts of Interest: The author declares no conflict of interest.

References

1. Brągoszewska, E.; Biedroń, I.; Mainka, A. Microbiological Air Quality in a Highschool Gym Located in an Urban Area of Southern Poland—Preliminary Research. *Atmosphere* **2020**, *11*, 797. [CrossRef]
2. Małecka-Adamowicz, M.; Koim-Puchowska, B.; Dembowska, E.A. Diversity of Bioaerosols in Selected Rooms of Two Schools and Antibiotic Resistance of Isolated Staphylococcal Strains (Bydgoszcz, Poland): A Case Study. *Atmosphere* **2020**, *11*, 1105. [CrossRef]
3. Zender-Świercz, E. Microclimate in Rooms Equipped with Decentralized Façade Ventilation Device. *Atmosphere* **2020**, *11*, 800. [CrossRef]
4. Skowron, K.; Grudlewska-Buda, K.; Kożuszko, S.; Wiktorczyk, N.; Skowron, K.J.; Mikucka, A.; Bernaciak, Z.; Gospodarek-Komkowska, E. Efficacy of Radiant Catalytic Ionization in Reduction of *Enterococcus* spp., *Clostridioides difficile* and *Staphylococcus aureus* in Indoor Air. *Atmosphere* **2020**, *11*, 764. [CrossRef]
5. Brągoszewska, E.; Bogacka, M.; Pikoń, K. Effectiveness and Eco-Costs of Air Cleaners in Terms of Improving Fungal Air Pollution in Dwellings Located in Southern Poland—A Preliminary Study. *Atmosphere* **2020**, *11*, 1255. [CrossRef]

atmosphere

Article

Effectiveness and Eco-Costs of Air Cleaners in Terms of Improving Fungal Air Pollution in Dwellings Located in Southern Poland—A Preliminary Study

Ewa Brągoszewska *, Magdalena Bogacka and Krzysztof Pikoń

Department of Technologies and Installations for Waste Management, Faculty of Energy and Environmental Engineering, Silesian University of Technology, 18 Konarskiego St., 44-100 Gliwice, Poland; magdalena.bogacka@polsl.pl (M.B.); krzysztof.pikon@polsl.pl (K.P.)
* Correspondence: ewa.bragoszewska@polsl.pl

Received: 9 October 2020; Accepted: 19 November 2020; Published: 21 November 2020

Abstract: Epidemiological evidence shows that air pollution is responsible for several million premature deaths per year. By virtue of being responsible for these deaths, economic evidence shows that air pollution also imposes a so-called economic cost to society of several trillion dollars per year. The diseases caused by biological air pollutants are of primary global concern for both social and economic reasons, and given that people may spend more than 90% of their time in enclosed spaces, the investigation into methods to remove indoor air pollutants is of paramount importance. One of the methods to improve indoor air quality (IAQ) is to use air cleaners (ACLs) with high-efficiency particulate air filters (HEPA) that remove biological indoor air pollutants from indoor environments. This work presents the results of a study of fungal aerosol samples collected during the summer season from inside two dwellings (DG1 and DG2) before and after starting the use of ACLs. The fungal aerosol samples collected from each of the six stages of the sampler were incubated on agar plates at 26 °C, and the colony forming units (CFU) were manually counted and statistically corrected. The concentration of living airborne fungi was expressed as the CFU in the volume of air (CFU·m^{-3}). The average concentration of fungal aerosol decreased the most when the ACLs were active for 24 min. The reduction was from 474 CFU·m^{-3} to 306 CFU·m^{-3}, and from 582 CFU·m^{-3} to 338 CFU·m^{-3} in DG1 and DG2, respectively. The use of ACLs was assessed by the life cycle assessment (LCA) methodology. This study highlights the benefits of controlling biological air pollutants in order to keep occupants of buildings happy and healthy.

Keywords: biological air pollutants; fungal aerosol; air cleaner; life cycle assessment; indoor air quality

1. Introduction

With the ongoing improvements in quality of life, indoor air quality (IAQ) has become an area of concern for researchers in the last few decades [1]. People spend the majority of their time indoors, and lowering the indoor concentrations of air pollutants is fundamental for our health and wellbeing, while conserving energy in residential indoor environments [2]. In particular, poor IAQ can be harmful to vulnerable groups such as children, young adults, the elderly, or those suffering from chronic respiratory and/or cardiovascular diseases [3]. Therefore, the development of indoor air decontamination technologies is highly desirable [4–6].

In recent years, a growing number of studies have focused on the assessment of exposure to biological air pollutants in indoor spaces with respect to the various negative effects on human health [7,8]. Interest in exposure to biological air pollutants (e.g., bacteria, fungi, and viruses) has increased in the 21st century, because they are associated with a wide range of health problems with a major impact on public health. These health problems include infection by disease, acute toxic effects, allergies, and even cancer [9–12]. The spread of infectious is of worldwide concern for social and economic reasons, e.g., seasonal influenza kills 200–500 thousand people annually [13].

Among biological air pollutants, the particles of fungal aerosols may be transported into buildings on the surface of new materials or on clothing [14–17]. They may also penetrate buildings through active or passive ventilation [18,19]. Symptoms of tiredness and memory loss, as well as common diseases such as allergies, asthma, and hypersensitivity pneumonitis, are caused by fungal aerosol exposure [20–22]. Fungal diversity is enormous, with more than an estimated one million species that produce airborne spores, conidia, hyphae, and other fragments that can affect human health [23]. Almost 10% of people worldwide suffer from a fungal allergy [24]. Therefore, the reduction of exposure to indoor fungal aerosols represents a particular challenge.

Natural ventilation is a common method used in homes to remove harmful toxins that may arise from the activity of the occupants. Its zero-energy cost is also important. Nowadays, when outdoor air pollution is an increasing problem, HVAC (heating, ventilation, and air conditioning) systems are used more and more often, which help to obtain the appropriate quality of indoor air [25,26]. However, one of the major drawbacks in this case is the high energy cost of operating these systems [13]. As an intermediate solution, air cleaners (ACLs) are becoming more and more popular in households, the operation of which increases the energy cost to a lesser extent, and at the same time ensures cleaning of the internal air [27]. One of the common methods of air purification is filtration, and the materials commonly used are high efficiency particulate filters (HEPAs). The use of activated carbon filters is equally popular [28].

The American Household Appliances Association (AHAM) established an air purifier standard in 1984, describing the method used to test the particle removal efficiency of air filters [29]. Three key elements contribute to the efficiency of an air filter, namely: room size, clean air delivery rate (CADR), and particle size category. CADR is the product of the filter removal efficiency and the airflow rate through the device, experimentally determined as the difference between the decay constants with and without the ACL running, multiplied by the effective indoor mixing volume [30].

HEPA filters are typically constructed from two media choices—polytetrafluoroethylene (PTFE) membrane or micro glass fibers. The thickness of the media can play a large role in the filter operating performance [31]. As public awareness of air pollution increases, HEPA filters in ACLs are becoming widely used in Poland by the growing middle class. In an ACL, the air is forced through the HEPA filter and the particles are physically captured. The key mechanisms of this action are diffusion, interception, inertial impaction, and sieving [32]. Studies have shown that HEPA filters can reduce particle concentrations by more than 50% [4,33,34].

There is also some evidence to suggest that these reductions lead to improvements in cardiorespiratory health [35,36]. Moreover, studies have reported that the use of indoor ACLs may be associated with a reduction in blood pressure, oxidative stress, and systemic inflammation, and may also improve lung function [4]. Therefore, it is important to reduce and control the concentrations of harmful microorganisms in the air in order to ensure good IAQ [37]. However, contaminated HEPA filters serve as an ecological niche for indoor microorganisms [38,39]. Moreover, the bulky structure of the HEPA filter requires a large working space and causes a large pressure difference between the inlet and outlet of the filter, and limits the efficiency of the air circulation [39].

This study includes four aspects. Our main goal was to evaluate of the impact of ACLs on the fungal IAQ. Therefore, we investigated the concentration and size distribution of fungal aerosols in two dwellings located in Southern Poland. We also calculated the ecological cost of air purification using the life cycle assessment (LCA) technique.

2. Experiments

2.1. Sampling Sites

The study was carried out in two living rooms at two dwellings located in Bytom (18°54′ E 50°23′ N) in Southern Poland. Each analyzed living room was equipped with the same type of ACL, with a PET (polyester) pre-filter retaining larger air pollutants, HEPA-11 filter with an area of 2.2 m^2, and an adsorption filter with active carbon (an absorbing area of 57,000 m^2). The research was conducted over a period of two months during the summer season of 2020. The sampling was performed once a week. A sample was taken when the ACLs were turned off, and again 12 min and 24 min after the ACLs were turned on. Samples were collected between 16:00 p.m. and 18:00 p.m. in order to check the efficiency of the tested device. Three sets of measurements were performed in each living room with the ACL turned on and turned off. Samples of airborne fungi were collected from the center of each room at a height of about 1.5 m in order to simulate aspiration from the human breathing zone. Each sample included six impaction stages with Petri dishes. In total, 864 Petri dishes (without blanks) with biological material were analyzed during the study.

The measurement was conducted in two living rooms, each with a volume of approximately 64 m^3. The assessment of the effectiveness of the air decontamination was carried out in the natural conditions of the residents' routine activities. Each living room was equipped with an ACL, with a Clean Air Delivery Rate (CADR) of 310 m^3/h. The windows in the rooms were closed during the study, and the air change per hour (ACH) was 0. Table 1 presents a description of the analyzed dwellings.

Table 1. Environmental parameters (mean +/− standard deviation), and a basic description of dwellings.

Parameters and Basic Description of DG1 and DG2	Dwelling 1 (DG1)	Dwelling 2 (DG2)
Home localization	close the city center	close the city center
Building built-in	1990s	1980s
Equipment	table, chairs, sofa	table, chairs, sofa, 2 armchairs
Ventilation system	natural	natural
Volume, m^3	64	62
Number of occupants	4 (2 adults and 2 children)	4 (2 adults and 2 children)
Number of animals	-	2 dogs
Floor covered with	PVC and carpet	PVC and carpet
Indoor temperature, °C	22.5 +/− 5.1	20.5 +/− 4.4
Indoor relative humidity, %	41. +/− 8.1	48.2 +/− 3.9
Outdoor temperature, °C	29.1 +/− 4.2	28.6 +/− 3.3
Outdoor relative humidity, %	39.1 +/− 7.4	44.2 +/− 8.9

The scheme of an ACL is presented in Figure 1.

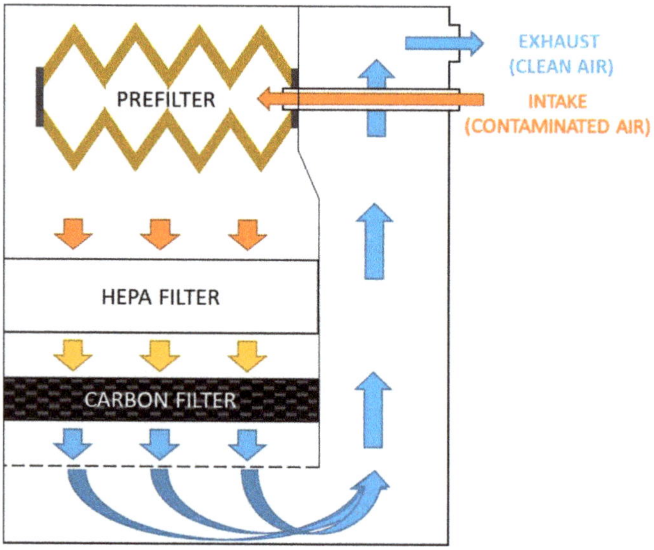

Figure 1. The scheme of typical filters used in the air cleaner (ACL) device.

2.2. Sampling and Analysis Methods

Measurements of the fungal aerosol concentrations were conducted using a six-stage Andersen impactor with cut-off diameters of 7.0, 4.7, 3.3, 2.1, 1.1, and 0.65 μm with an air flow of 28.3 dm^3/min, and the sampling time was 10 min (calculated following Nevalainen et al. [40]). For sampling the fungal particles, we used Petri dishes containing a solid nutrient medium located on all of the impactor stages. Malt extract agar (MEA 2%, Biocorp, Warsaw, Poland) culture media with chloramphenicol was used to speciate the fungal aerosol. The samples were incubated for five to six days at 26 °C. The concentration of living microorganisms was counted as the number of colony forming units in the volume of air ($CFU \cdot m^{-3}$).

According to our previous studies [41,42], the quality control procedure was practiced using PN-EN12322 [43] and ISO 11133:2014 [44] standards.

2.3. Statistical Analysis

Based on the Shapiro–Wilk test results, it was found that all of the samples had a normal distribution in terms of the tested parameters. Student's t-test ($p < 0.05$) was used to detect the presence of a statistically significant difference between when the ACL was turned off (ACLO) and the samples when the air cleaner was active (ACLA) for 12 min and 24 min. The statistical analysis was performed using Statistica v.12.

2.4. LCA Methodology

In an environmental analysis, many LCA methodologies are used. One LCA methodology practiced here was ReCiPe 2008, with the same operation details as in our previous studies [41]. The next part of the analysis was the environmental aspect. In order to calculate the impact on the environment, the analysis should follow the ISO 14040: 2006 standard [45]. This methodology is based on the full life cycle, which includes three main stages, namely: production, use, and disposal. Figure 2 presents the phases in the case of air ventilation linked with purification in terms of reducing fungal air pollution in dwellings. Depending on the individual case, the description of these phases should be more precise. The LCA includes transportation, different waste scenarios, and so on. In order to assess the real impact, the analysis should include all materials, pollution, and consumption involved in making the product. LCA is based on assumptions and it reveals the most important negative inputs or outputs [46,47]. In this study, the analysis was conducted using SimaPro software with the Ecoinvent 3.0 database. The results are given as percentages so as to visualize the impact of each of the phases in the complete analysis.

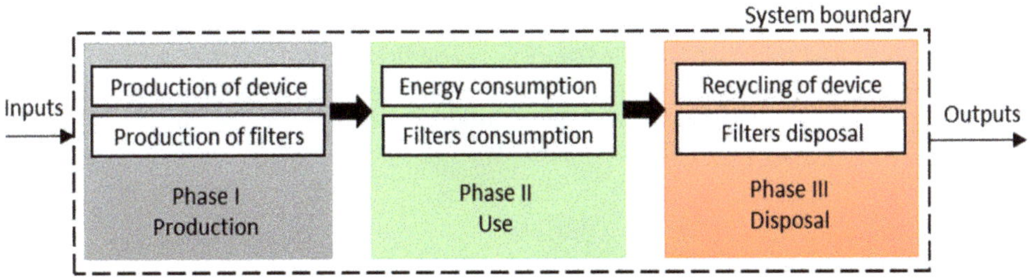

Figure 2. The scheme of life cycle assessment (LCA) phases in the process of air cleaning.

3. Results and Discussion

3.1. The Concentration of Culturable Fungal Aerosol and the Effectiveness of ACLs

The average concentrations of airborne fungi collected from the indoor air are presented in Table 2. The average concentration of fungal aerosols significantly ($p < 0.01$) decreased when the ACL was active for 24 min, from 474 CFU·m^{-3} to 306 CFU·m^{-3}, and from 582 CFU·m^{-3} to 338 CFU·m^{-3} in DG1 and DG2, respectively. So, the reduction of fungal aerosols was 35% in DG1 and 42% in DG2. In the case of the average concentration of culturable fungal spores when the ACL was active for 12 min, in DG1 we observed a decrease from 474 CFU·m^{-3} (ACLO) to 373 CFU·m^{-3} with a significant difference ($p = 0.04$), while in DG2 with the same operation time for the ACL, we observed a decrease from 582 CFU·m^{-3} (ACLO) to 419 CFU·m^{-3} ($p < 0.01$). The reduction of fungal particles after 12 min of ACL operation was 21% and 28% in DG1 and DG2, respectively. Both times of purification proved to be effective for the removal of fungal aerosols. However, the reduction of fungal aerosols was more effective after the extended use of the air cleaner.

The results obtained in our study correspond with our earlier research in which we determined the effect of ACLs in eliminating bacterial microorganisms; when ACLs were enabled, the concentration of bacterial aerosols was reduced by about 50% [41]. Similar studies conducted in central Poland indicate that the effectiveness of filters in air decontamination in nursery schools is 41% [48]. However, the ACL is only effective during the operation period; it does not eliminate sources of fungal contamination. ACLs do not provide a fundamental solution to fungal contamination [49].

Table 2. Average concentration and standard deviation (SD) of fungal aerosol colony-forming units per cubic meter of air (CFU·m^{-3}) inside two types of dwellings: dwelling 1 (DG1) and dwelling 2 (DG2), when the air cleaner was active (ACLA) for 12 min and 24 min, or when the air cleaner was turn off (ACLO).

Location	Average Concentration CFU·m^{-3} +/−SD	Minimum	Maximum
DG1 ACLA/12 min	373 +/− 101	21	410
DG2 ACLA/12 min	419 +/−124	14	544
DG1 ACLA/24 min	306 +/−92	18	404
DG2 ACLA/24 min	338 +/−86	4	419
DG1 ACLO	474 +/−134	14	522
DG2 ACLO	582 +/−141	7	640

Moreover, under the current COVID-19 pandemic situation, ACLs could be used as a supplementary and precautionary method after other more significant activities have been taken, such as local source control, frequent disinfection of the room and furnishing surfaces, and ventilation [50].

3.2. The Size Distribution of Fungal Aerosol and the Effectiveness of ACLs

The mean distributions of the aerodynamic diameters of the airborne fungi are shown in Figure 3. It can be seen that the size distribution of fungi when the air cleaner was turned off (ACLO) in the analyzed dwellings was characterized by a large share of particles in an aerodynamic diameter (d_{ae}) range of 2.1–3.3 μm. Aerosols smaller than 5 μm in the aerodynamic diameter contribute to airborne infection [51]. An increase in the share of the coarser fraction of airborne fungi when the air cleaner was active (ACLA) may be as a result of the reemission process generated by the air blowing from ACLs.

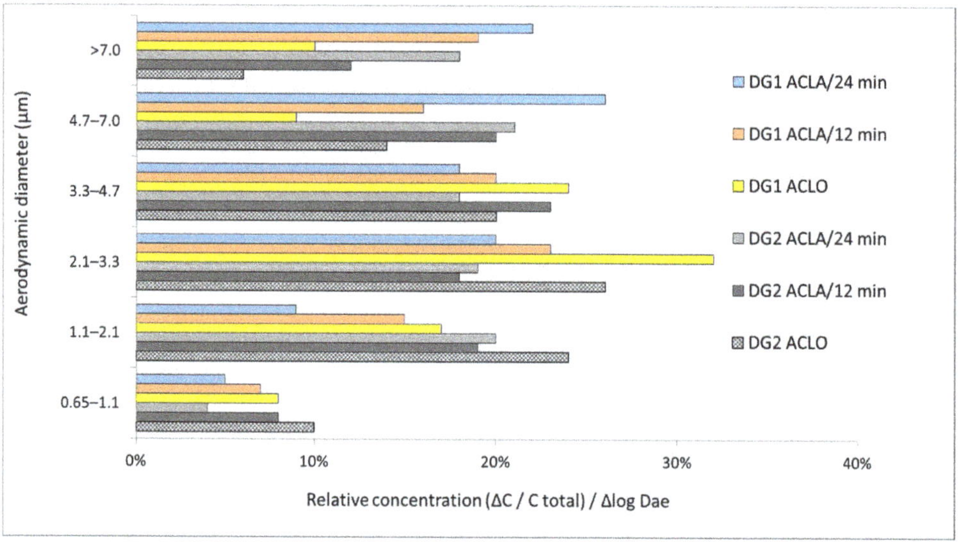

Figure 3. The size distribution of fungal aerosols in dwelling 1 (DG1) and dwelling 2 (DG2) when the air cleaner was active (ACLA) for 12 min and 24 min, or when the air cleaner was turned off (ACLO).

We observed that while the air cleaner was active (ACLA), the respirable fraction of analyzed bioaerosol (particles less than 3.3 μm) decreased compared with the results when the air cleaner was turned off (ACLO) in DG1 by approximately 13% and 19%, and decreased in DG2 by approximately 15% and 17% when the ACLA for 12 min and 24 min, respectively.

The HEPA filters built into ACLs are made of intertwined fibers, where the smallest particles or bioaerosols become retained in three ways, namely: interception, impaction, or diffusion. The fine fraction of biological particles are most likely trapped in the fibers by means of diffusion [29].

Exposure of residents to respirable fungal particles may result not only in infections related directly to contact with microbial pathogens, but may also cause diseases associated with the exposure to mycotoxins and fungal glucans [52]. The symptoms caused by exposure to a fraction of fungal particles less than 3.3 μm include bronchitis, allergic asthma, obstructive pulmonary disease, alveolitis, or organic dust toxic syndrome [53].

Fungal aerosols do not grow well indoors if there is insufficient water and moisture in the materials and substrates. The current recommended procedures for controlling indoor fungal growth in the dwelling are to stop and control all moisture and water problems, remove contaminated materials under containment so as to avoid the dispersal of fungal spores, and the use of HEPA filters in indoor environments [54].

There is a still lack of global standards and guidelines for microbiological indoor air quality. Therefore, measurements of indoor bioaerosols should be conducted much more intensely and on a larger scale. Portable and affordable ACLs have the potential to reduce the exposure of people to bioaerosols in indoor environments, but further work is needed, particularly focused on the reemission process generated by the air blowing from ACLs. The elucidation of this relationship will be an important foundation from which to develop air cleaning technologies.

3.3. LCA—The Ecological Cost of Emission Reduction

Table 3 presents a list of assumptions based on the Ecoinvent database. It shows the complex data that should be included, but with some limitations due to a lack in the database. Regarding the LCA phases, the three main phases are production, use, and disposal.

Table 3. Assumptions for LCA of air cleaning.

LCA	Product/Service	Assumption	Unit	Chosen Ecoinvent Database
Phase I Production	Production of the device	1	piece	Air filter, decentralized unit, 180–250 m^3/h {RER}| production | Alloc Def, U
	Production of the carbon filter	1	piece	Included in device production
	Production of the HEPA filter	1	piece	Included in device production
Phase II Use	Electricity consumption	85.5	kWh/year	Electricity, low voltage {PL}| market for | Alloc Def, U
	Filter changes	1	piece/year	Not included (for the first year the original filter is used)
Phase III Disposal	Recycling of plastic	2	kg	_42 Recycling of plastics basic, EU27
	Recycling of metal	1	kg	_60 Recycling of metals basic, n.e.c., EU27
	Disposal of filters	1	kg	Not included (lack of database)

Of course, in the disposal phase, only recycling options are presented, but more scenarios can be predicted like the landfill or a scenario where only half of the materials will be recycled. However, regarding the regulations of the Waste Electrical and Electronic Equipment Directive (WEEE) [55], it should be collected by dedicated companies, and because of this, this scenario is presented as the most probable. In the article, the LCA analysis should show the main value of LCA and that everything has an impact on the environment; even people who think about our health and that it is the most important issue, we always have an impact on the environment. In other scenarios, we can predict that the impact on the environment will be higher than what is presented. The analysis was based on SimarPro software. The results are presented in Figure 4.

In each category, the "use phase" has the biggest impact on the environment. Taking into account the assumption that metals and plastics are recycled at the end of the life of the device, in each category, the impact is negative, which means that it has positive results, particularly when linked to the replacement effect. The impact of the production of the device is less than 1% per category. The main conclusion is that the impact of cleaning air is mostly associated with electricity consumption. For the test carried out in Poland, the electricity mix comes from coal, and therefore its impact is huge. If it is compared with the environmental impact of another electricity mix, for example in France, the total impact will be much lower.

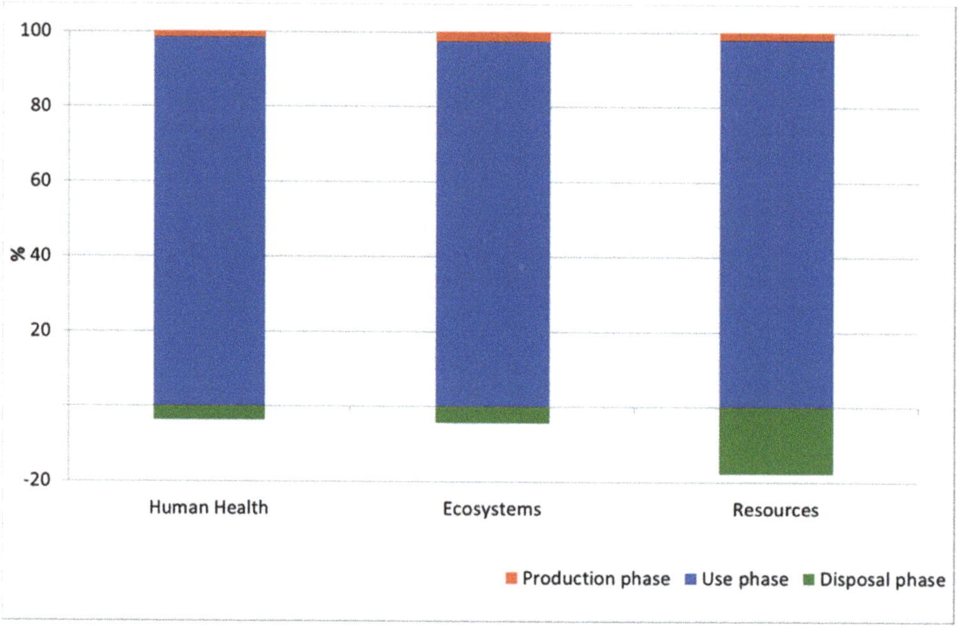

Figure 4. The LCA analysis of ReCiPe Endpoint (H) and the damage assessment in %.

Environmental impact is a very important issue that could be treated as a form of external cost, which is currently high on the agenda and should be taken into account in order to deliver a better picture of the processes under analysis. This is not a question of whether or not should we sacrifice human health for a lower carbon footprint. It is rather a question of a more holistic view that would lead to more informed decisions and better scientific credibility. LCA is very important in every field. Like economic analysis, each measure should be calculated and analyzed as broadly as possible. LCA analysis allows us to assess the impact on the environment, but also on human health in the full life cycle, i.e., from the extraction of natural resources, through production, transport, use, and management. During this analysis, the real results on the environment and human health can be predicted, taking into account all of the stages and the many dimensions of the problem, and not only the benefits of using certain products. The article presents this problem more generally because the aim of the article is to present the research and results of the removal of fungi from the air. However, the LCA can indicate that this also affects the environment and human health in another dimension.

4. Conclusions

A study of the quantity of fungal aerosols and the ecological cost of pollution reduction was carried out in dwellings in Southern Poland during the summer season. Although the presented research is the result of preliminary studies, it allows for the following conclusions to be drawn.

Air purification has an impact on the environment. Electricity and materials, including chemicals, are needed in almost every process, but this cost is much lower than the cost of contaminated air on health. This problem is also linked with waste; the filters are contaminated with pollutants and should be disposed of with special care.

In our study, both analyzed of the times of purification (12 min and 24 min) proved to be effective for the removal of fungal aerosols. However, the reduction in the average concentration of fungal aerosols was more effective after an extended use of air cleaners.

The current findings suggest the need for further work, particularly focused on a reemission process generated by air blowing from ACLs. The elucidation of this relationship will be an important foundation from which to develop air cleaning technologies.

Microbial pollution is one of the most fundamental indoor environmental quality problems indoors. Therefore, we believe that our study will point out the need for implementing a strategy to control and improve microbiological air quality in indoor environments.

Author Contributions: Conceptualization, E.B.; data curation, E.B. and M.B.; methodology, E.B. and M.B.; supervision, K.P.; visualization, E.B.; writing—original draft, E.B. and M.B.; writing—review and editing, E.B., M.B. and K.P. All authors have read and agreed to the published version of the manuscript.

Funding: Research funded by subsidies granted for the year 2019 from the Department of Technology and Installations for Waste Management, Silesian University of Technology (grant number 08/030/BKM20/0081).

Conflicts of Interest: The authors declare no conflict of interest.

References

1. Saini, J.; Dutta, M.; Marques, G. A comprehensive review on indoor air quality monitoring systems for enhanced public health. *Sustain. Environ. Res.* **2020**, *30*, 1–12. [CrossRef]
2. Simoni, M.; Jaakkola, M.S.; Carrozzi, L.; Baldacci, S.; Di Pede, F.; Viegi, G. Indoor air pollution and respiratory health in the elderly. *Eur. Respir. J.* **2003**, *21*, 15S–20S. [CrossRef]
3. Cincinelli, A.; Martellini, T.; Cincinelli, A.; Martellini, T. Indoor Air Quality and Health. *Int. J. Environ. Res. Public Health* **2017**, *14*, 1286. [CrossRef] [PubMed]
4. Kelly, F.J.; Fussell, J.C. Improving indoor air quality, health and performance within environments where people live, travel, learn and work. *Atmos. Environ.* **2019**, *200*, 90–109. [CrossRef]
5. Yang, Y.; Zhang, B.; Feng, Q.; Cai, H.; Jiang, M.; Zhou, K.; Li, F.; Liu, S.; Li, X. Towards locating time-varying indoor particle sources: Development of two multi-robot olfaction methods based on whale optimization algorithm. *Build. Environ.* **2019**, *166*, 106413. [CrossRef]
6. Brauer, M.; Hoek, G.; Smit, H.A.; De Jongste, J.C.; Gerritsen, J.; Postma, D.S.; Kerkhof, M.; Brunekreef, B. Air pollution and development of asthma, allergy and infections in a birth cohort. *Eur. Respir. J.* **2007**, *29*, 879–888. [CrossRef] [PubMed]
7. Qian, J.; Hospodsky, D.; Yamamoto, N.; Nazaroff, W.W.; Peccia, J. Size-resolved emission rates of airborne bacteria and fungi in an occupied classroom. *Indoor Air* **2012**, *22*, 339–351. [CrossRef] [PubMed]
8. Van Leuken, J.P.G.; Swart, A.N.; Droogers, P.; Van Pul, A.; Heederik, D.; Havelaar, A.H. Climate change effects on airborne pathogenic bioaerosol concentrations: A scenario analysis. *Aerobiologia* **2016**, *32*, 607–617. [CrossRef] [PubMed]
9. Fröhlich-Nowoisky, J.; Kampf, C.J.; Weber, B.; Huffman, J.A.; Pöhlker, C.; Andreae, M.O.; Lang-Yona, N.; Burrows, S.M.; Gunthe, S.S.; Elbert, W.; et al. Bioaerosols in the Earth system: Climate, health, and ecosystem interactions. *Atmos. Res.* **2016**, *182*, 346–376. [CrossRef]
10. Reinmuth-Selzle, K.; Kampf, C.J.; Lucas, K.; Lang-Yona, N.; Fröhlich-Nowoisky, J.; Shiraiwa, M.; Lakey, P.S.J.; Lai, S.; Liu, F.; Kunert, A.T.; et al. Air Pollution and Climate Change Effects on Allergies in the Anthropocene: Abundance, Interaction, and Modification of Allergens and Adjuvants. *Environ. Sci. Technol.* **2017**, *51*, 4119–4141. [CrossRef]
11. Samake, A.; Uzu, G.; Martins, J.M.F.; Calas, A.; Vince, E.; Parat, S.; Jaffrezo, J.L. The unexpected role of bioaerosols in the Oxidative Potential of PM. *Sci. Rep.* **2017**, *7*, 1–10. [CrossRef] [PubMed]
12. Kim, K.-H.; Kabir, E.; Jahan, S.A. Airborne bioaerosols and their impact on human health. *J. Environ. Sci.* **2018**, *67*, 23–35. [CrossRef] [PubMed]
13. Aliabadi, A.A.; Rogak, S.N.; Bartlett, K.H.; Green, S.I. Preventing Airborne Disease Transmission: Review of Methods for Ventilation Design in Health Care Facilities. *Adv. Prev. Med.* **2011**, *2011*, 1–21. [CrossRef] [PubMed]
14. Kildesø, J.; Würtz, H.; Nielsen, K.F.; Kruse, P.; Wilkins, K.; Thrane, U.; Gravesen, S.; Nielsen, P.A.; Schneider, T. Determination of fungal spore release from wet building materials. *Indoor Air* **2003**, *13*, 148–155. [CrossRef]
15. Li, D.-W.; Yang, C.S. Fungal Contamination as a Major Contributor to Sick Building Syndrome. *Adv. Appl. Microbiol.* **2004**, *55*, 31–112. [CrossRef]

16. Kulkarni, P.; Baron, P.; Willeke, K. *Aerosol Measurement: Principles, Techniques, and Applications*, 3rd ed.; Wiley: Hoboken, NJ, USA, 2011.
17. Shelton, B.G.; Kirkland, K.H.; Flanders, W.D.; Morris, G.K. Profiles of airborne fungi in buildings and outdoor environments in the United States. *Appl. Environ. Microbiol.* **2002**, *68*, 1743–1753. [CrossRef]
18. WHO. *Guidelines for Indoor Air Quality: Dampness and Mould*; WHO Regional Office for Europe: Copenhagen, Denmark, 2009; ISBN 7989289041683.
19. Ghosh, B.; Lal, H.; Srivastava, A. Review of bioaerosols in indoor environment with special reference to sampling, analysis and control mechanisms. *Environ. Int.* **2015**, *85*, 254–272. [CrossRef]
20. King, M.D.; Lacey, R.E.; Pak, H.; Fearing, A.; Ramos, G.; Baig, T.; Smith, B.; Koustova, A. Assays and enumeration of bioaerosols-traditional approaches to modern practices. *Aerosol Sci. Technol.* **2020**, *54*, 611–633. [CrossRef]
21. Siersted, H.C.; Gravesen, S. Extrinsic allergic alveolitis after exposure to the yeast Rhodotorula rubra. *Allergy* **1993**, *48*, 298–299. [CrossRef]
22. Selman, M.; Lacasse, Y.; Pardo, A.; Cormier, Y. Hypersensitivity Pneumonitis Caused by Fungi. *Proc. Am. Thorac. Soc.* **2010**, *7*, 229–236. [CrossRef]
23. Lee, J.H.; Hwang, G.B.; Jung, J.H.; Lee, D.H.; Lee, B.U. Generation characteristics of fungal spore and fragment bioaerosols by airflow control over fungal cultures. *J. Aerosol Sci.* **2010**, *41*, 319–325. [CrossRef]
24. Yassin, M.F.; Almouqatea, S. Assessment of airborne bacteria and fungi in an indoor and outdoor environment. *Int. J. Environ. Sci. Technol.* **2010**, *7*, 535–544. [CrossRef]
25. Liu, Z.J.; Ma, S.Y.; Cao, G.Q.; Meng, C.; He, B.J. Distribution characteristics, growth, reproduction andtransmission modes and control strategies for microbial contamination in HVAC systems: A literature review. *Energy Build.* **2018**, *177*, 77–95. [CrossRef]
26. Liu, Z.; Zhu, Z.; Zhu, Y.; Xu, W.; Li, H. Investigation of dust loading and culturable microorganisms of HVAC systems in 24 office buildings in Beijing. *Energy Build.* **2015**, *103*, 166–174. [CrossRef]
27. Cheng, K.-C.; Park, H.-K.; Tetteh, A.O.; Zheng, D.; Ouellette, N.T.; Nadeau, K.C.; Hildemann, L.M. Mixing and sink effects of air purifiers on indoor PM2.5 concentrations: A pilot study of eight residential homes in Fresno, California. *Aerosol Sci. Technol.* **2016**, *50*, 835–845. [CrossRef]
28. Gunschera, J.; Markewitz, D.; Bansen, B.; Salthammer, T.; Ding, H. Portable photocatalytic air cleaners: efficiencies and by-product generation. *Environ. Sci. Pollut. Res.* **2016**, *23*, 7482–7493. [CrossRef] [PubMed]
29. Lee, J.H.; Kim, J.Y.; Cho, B.-B.; Anusha, J.R.; Sim, J.Y.; Raj, C.J.; Yu, K.-H. Assessment of air purifier on efficient removal of airborne bacteria, Staphylococcus epidermidis, using single-chamber method. *Environ. Monit. Assess.* **2019**, *191*, 720. [CrossRef]
30. Shaughnessy, R.J.; Sextro, R.G. What Is an Effective Portable Air Cleaning Device? A Review. *J. Occup. Environ. Hyg.* **2006**, *3*, 169–181. [CrossRef]
31. Hiner, S. Not all HEPA filters are the same. *Power Eng.* **2017**, *121*, 5.
32. Yang, C. Aerosol Filtration Application Using Fibrous Media—An Industrial Perspective. *Chin. J. Chem. Eng.* **2012**, *20*, 1–9. [CrossRef]
33. Batterman, S.; Du, L.; Mentz, G.; Mukherjee, B.; Parker, E.; Godwin, C.; Chin, J.-Y.; O'Toole, A.; Robins, T.; Rowe, Z.; et al. Particulate matter concentrations in residences: An intervention study evaluating stand-alone filters and air conditioners. *Indoor Air* **2012**, *22*, 235–252. [CrossRef] [PubMed]
34. Wheeler, A.J.; Gibson, M.D.; MacNeill, M.; Ward, T.J.; Wallace, L.A.; Kuchta, J.; Seaboyer, M.; Dabek-Zlotorzynska, E.; Guernsey, J.R.; Stieb, D.M. Impacts of Air Cleaners on Indoor Air Quality in Residences Impacted by Wood Smoke. *Environ. Sci. Technol.* **2014**, *48*, 12157–12163. [CrossRef] [PubMed]
35. Fisk, W.J. Health benefits of particle filtration. *Indoor Air* **2013**, *23*, 357–368. [CrossRef] [PubMed]
36. Morishita, M.; Thompson, K.C.; Brook, R.D. Understanding Air Pollution and Cardiovascular Diseases: Is It Preventable? *Curr. Cardiovasc. Risk Rep.* **2015**, *9*, 1–9. [CrossRef]
37. Onmek, N.; Kongcharoen, J.; Singtong, A.; Penjumrus, A.; Junnoo, S. Environmental Factors and Ventilation Affect Concentrations of Microorganisms in Hospital Wards of Southern Thailand. *J. Environ. Public Health* **2020**, *2020*, 1–8. [CrossRef]
38. Guo, J.; Xiong, Y.; Kang, T.; Xiang, Z.; Qin, C. Bacterial community analysis of floor dust and HEPA filters in air purifiers used in office rooms in ILAS, Beijing. *Sci. Rep.* **2020**, *10*, 1–11. [CrossRef]

39. Choi, S.-J.; Kim, K.H.; Kim, H.J.; Yoon, J.S.; Lee, M.J.; Choi, K.-S.; Sung, U.-D.; Park, W.-T.; Lee, J.; Jeon, J.; et al. Highly Efficient, Flexible, and Recyclable Air Filters Using Polyimide Films with Patterned Thru-Holes Fabricated by Ion Milling. *Appl. Sci.* **2019**, *9*, 235. [CrossRef]
40. Nevalainen, A.; Willeke, K.; Liebhaber, F.; Pastuszka, J.S.; Burge, H.; Henningson, E. Bioaerosol sampling. In *Aerosol Measurement: Principles, Techniques and Applications*; Willeke, K., Baron, P., Eds.; Van Nostrand Reinhold: New York, NY, USA, 1993; pp. 471–492.
41. Brągoszewska, E.; Bogacka, M.; Pikoń, K. Efficiency and Eco-Costs of Air Purifiers in Terms of Improving Microbiological Indoor Air Quality in Dwellings—A Case Study. *Atmosphere* **2019**, *10*, 742. [CrossRef]
42. Brągoszewska, E.; Biedroń, I. Indoor Air Quality and Potential Health Risk Impacts of Exposure to Antibiotic Resistant Bacteria in an Office Rooms in Southern Poland. *Int. J. Environ. Res. Public Health* **2018**, *15*, 2604. [CrossRef]
43. PN-EN 12322 In Vitro Diagnostic Medical Devices. Culture Media for Microbiology. Performance Criteria for Culture Media. 2005. Available online: https://ec.europa.eu/growth/single-market/european-standards/harmonised-standards/iv-diagnostic-medical-devices_en (accessed on 1 October 2020).
44. ISO 11133 Microbiology of Food, Animal Feed and Water—Preparation, Production, Storage and Performance Testing of Culture Media. 2014. Available online: https://www.iso.org/standard/53610.html (accessed on 1 October 2020).
45. *Environmental Management—Life Cycle Assessment—Principles and Framework*; ISO 14040; International Organization for Standardization (ISO): Geneva, Switzerland, 2006.
46. Bogacka, M.; Pikoń, K. Best Practice In Environmental Impact Evaluation Based On Lca—Methodologies Review. In Proceedings of the 14th International Multidisciplinary Scientific GeoConference-SGEM, Albena, Bulgaria, 17–26 June 2014.
47. Pikoń, K.; Bogacka, M. Local Specificity in Environmental Impact Assessment—End-Point Local Evaluation Indicators. In Proceedings of the 14th International Multidisciplinary Scientific GeoConference-SGEM, Albena, Bulgaria, 17–26 June 2014.
48. Gayer, A.; Mucha, D.; Adamkiewicz, Ł.; Badyda, A. Children exposure to PM2.5 in kindergarten classrooms equipped with air purifiers—A pilot study. In Proceedings of the International Conference on Fire and Environmental Safety Engineering (FESE 2018), Lviv, Ukraine, 7–8 November 2018.
49. Hashimoto, K.; Kawakami, Y. Effectiveness of Airborne Fungi Removal by using a HEPA Air Purifier Fan in Houses. *Biocontrol Sci.* **2018**, *23*, 215–221. [CrossRef]
50. Zhao, B.; Liu, Y.; Chen, C. Air purifiers: A supplementary measure to remove airborne SARS-CoV-2. *Build. Environ.* **2020**, *177*, 106918. [CrossRef] [PubMed]
51. Tellier, R. Aerosol transmission of influenza A virus: A review of new studies. *J. R. Soc. Interface* **2009**, *6*, S783–S790. [CrossRef] [PubMed]
52. Lacey, J.; Dutkiewicz, J. Bioaerosols and occupational lung disease. *J. Aerosol Sci.* **1994**, *25*, 1371–1404. [CrossRef]
53. Owen, M.; Ensor, D.; Sparks, L. Airborne particle sizes and sources found in indoor air. *Atmos. Environ. Part A Gen. Top.* **1992**, *26*, 2149–2162. [CrossRef]
54. Institute of Medicine. *Damp Indoor Spaces and Health*; The National Academies Press: Washington, DC, USA, 2004; ISBN 10-0-309-09193-4.
55. European Parliament and the Council of the European Union. Directive 2012/19/EU of 4 July 2012 on Waste Electrical and Electronic Equipment (WEEE). *Off. J. Eur. Union* **2012**, *55*, 38–71. Available online: http://eur-lex.europa.eu/ (accessed on 14 November 2020).

Publisher's Note: MDPI stays neutral with regard to jurisdictional claims in published maps and institutional affiliations.

atmosphere MDPI

Article

Diversity of Bioaerosols in Selected Rooms of Two Schools and Antibiotic Resistance of Isolated Staphylococcal Strains (Bydgoszcz, Poland): A Case Study

Marta Małecka-Adamowicz [1], Beata Koim-Puchowska [2] and Ewa A. Dembowska [1,*]

[1] Department of Microbiology and Immunobiology, Faculty of Biological Sciences, Kazimierz Wielki University, ul. Al. Powstańców Wielkopolskich 10, 85-090 Bydgoszcz, Poland; marmal@ukw.edu.pl
[2] Department of Biotechnology, Faculty of Biological Sciences, Kazimierz Wielki University, ul. Poniatowskiego12, 85-090 Bydgoszcz, Poland; koimpuch@ukw.edu.pl
* Correspondence: dembow@ukw.edu.pl; Tel.: +48-52-376-79-27

Received: 18 September 2020; Accepted: 13 October 2020; Published: 15 October 2020

Abstract: The present study is aimed at evaluating microbiological air pollution in libraries, cafeterias and selected classrooms of two schools in Bydgoszcz city, northern Poland and determining the antibiotic resistance of Staphylococcal strains isolated from the indoor air. One of the investigated schools (School A) is located in the very center of the city, in the vicinity of a park, among old houses and stone-lined streets, while the other (School B), among modern residential buildings, close to a street with heavy traffic. In each school, air samples were collected in the morning, always from all three sampling sites, using the MAS-100 sampler. Selective growth media were used for bacteria and mold isolation and quantifying analysis. The antibiotic resistance of the isolated mannitol-positive staphylococci was assessed using the disc diffusion method in accordance with EUCAST recommendations. The highest mean concentration of heterotrophic bacteria was recorded in the cafeterias: 884 CFU m^{-3} in School A and 1906 CFU m^{-3} in School B. Molds were the most abundant in the library and cafeteria in School B, where their average concentration exceeded 300 CFU m^{-3}. *Cladosporium* and *Penicillium* species prevailed, while *Fusarium*, *Acremonium* and *Aspergillus* were less abundant. Airborne mannitol-positive staphylococci were recorded at low concentrations, ranging from 6 to 11 CFU m^{-3} on average. According to the taxonomic analysis, *Staphylococcus aureus* isolates were the most abundant in both schools, followed by *S. xylosus*, *S. haemolyticus* and *S. saprophyticus*. The antibiograms indicated that resistance to erythromycin was common in 62.5% of the isolated staphylococcal strains. Levofloxacin and gentamicin were the most effective antibiotics. No multidrug-resistant strains were identified.

Keywords: indoor air quality; microbiological contamination; heterotrophic bacteria; antimicrobial resistance; mannitol-positive staphylococci; fungi

1. Introduction

Air quality in public facilities, including schools, is of growing concern. Numerous reports indicate that indoor air pollution is worse than outdoor air pollution and that the composition of indoor air microflora is more stable [1,2]. Although the concentrations of the majority of indoor air pollutants are so low that they cannot be considered harmful, long-term exposure may have negative effects on human health [3].

Indoor air contaminants come from different sources. Some of them, such as building materials, furnishings, ventilation systems and household products (e.g., air fresheners) can release pollutants almost continuously. Other sources, related to activities, such as smoking, cleaning or redecorating, release pollutants occasionally [4]. According to Andualem et al. [5] overcrowded classrooms, inadequate fresh air supply, poor construction and maintenance of school buildings negatively affect air quality in schools. Since students and teachers spend most of their day inside school buildings, the concentration of airborne microorganisms is an important parameter with a large impact on their performance, mental health and even physical condition [6]. Moreover, the absence of a student due to health issues may affect their academic achievements [7,8].

Particulate matter is considered an air pollutant of the greatest concern mainly due to its acute and chronic effects on children's health [9]. According to Du et al. [10] bacterial and fungal particles (PM 2.5) significantly affect air quality, contributing to the spread of infectious diseases and allergies [11]. Asthma is common in children with allergies. Since children spend most of their time in school, indoor air contamination can affect their pulmonary health [12].

The condition of educational facilities is a global problem because exposure to indoor air of poor quality may affect children's respiratory and cardiovascular functions [13], particularly since they breathe in more air in relation to their body weight than adults [14] and their immune system and internal organs are not yet fully developed [15]. In addition, young (and still growing) organisms are more susceptible to damage than mature ones [8]. Therefore, in institutions with an increased risk of pathogenic microbiota development, there is a need for monitoring air quality and evaluating the ability of pathogenic bacteria to acquire antibiotic resistance. According to Labi et al. [16] multidrug-resistant strains pose a serious threat to human health and are a challenge for modern medicine.

Ensuring good air quality in schools is of paramount importance for work efficiency, good health and mental wellbeing [17] and, as stated in WHO recommendations, access to air of acceptable quality is a fundamental human right.

In the available literature, there are numerous reports on air quality in classrooms in countries all over the world. However, since this type of research had been conducted only in the southern and central Poland prior to this study, the authors decided to investigate microbiological air contamination in schools in Bydgoszcz, the city located in northern Poland. Air samples were collected not only from classrooms (standard approach) but also from libraries and cafeterias. The analyses focused on three aspects. The main objective was to determine bioaerosol abundance in selected rooms and the influence of several factors (e.g., room type, room size, room temperature and season) on the concentration of individual microbial groups. Another objective was to determine the genera of microorganisms and their taxonomic affiliation. Finally, antibiotic resistance profiles of opportunistic staphylococci were prepared.

Based on the above objectives, the following hypotheses were formulated:

- The number of microbial groups is higher in smaller rooms and differs depending on the month of sampling;
- Room temperature affects the concentration of microorganisms;
- Opportunistic multidrug-resistant staphylococci are found in the air of the investigated school rooms.

2. Experiments

2.1. Sampling and Sampling Sites

Microbiological tests were carried out in two schools in Bydgoszcz City, Poland. School A is located in the city center, in the vicinity of a park, old residential buildings and cobbled streets, while School B is located among modern blocks of flats in a street with heavy traffic.

Air samples were collected in three parallel repetitions once a month from September to February in two schools (School A and School B) from three sampling sites in each school: I—classroom; II—library; III—cafeteria (Table 1). During each sample collection (always in the morning hours), the schools were open and filled with students.

Air (in the amount of 100 L) was collected 1.5 m above the ground with an MAS-100 sampler (Merck, Germany) with a dual-flow turbofan, which sucks the air stream through a metal head with 400 × 1 mm holes and directs it onto the surface of a sterile Petri dish with the substrate. A centrifugal fan, controlled by a flow sensor, regulates the air flow. The flow rate was 100 L per minute.

Samples were transported to the laboratory, placed in a thermostat and incubated for a specific time at an appropriate temperature. After that, grown colonies were counted. The results were corrected using the table of statistical corrections according to Feller [18] and expressed as colony-forming units per cubic meter of air (CFU m^{-3}).

Table 1. Description of sampling sites.

School Characteristics	**School A**			**School B**		
School location	53°07′37.3″ N 18°00′23.6″ E			53°06′38.1″ N 18°02′53.3″ E		
Year of construction	1878			1955		
Floor covering	Vinyl PCV, tiles			Vinyl PCV, tiles		
Number of children	760			600		
Age of children	14–19			14–19		
Sampling Site Characteristics	**School A**			**School B**		
	Classroom	**Library**	**Cafeteria**	**Classroom**	**Library**	**Cafeteria**
Sampling site location	Ground floor	First floor	Ground floor	Ground floor	Basement	Ground floor
Ventilation system	Natural	Natural	Natural, gravity	Natural	Natural	Natural, gravity
Surface area, m^2	45	83	14	48	72	20
Indoor temperature, °C (average)	23	22	23	22	22	22

2.2. Microbial Research

The total concentration of heterotrophic bacteria was determined using Trypticase Soy Lab Agar medium (BTL, Poland). The bacteria were incubated at 37 °C for 48 h; then, grown colonies were counted and their concentration was expressed as colony-forming units per cubic meter of air (CFU m^{-3}).

The presence of mannitol-positive staphylococci was detected using Chapman's nutrient medium (BTL, Poland). Bacterial cultures were incubated at 37 °C for 48 h; then, grown colonies were counted. Bright yellow zones around a grown colony indicated a positive result. Additionally, the strains were Gram stained and identified by as Gram-positive cocci. Taxonomic analysis of the strains was performed using API tests (API Staph bioMerieux, Craponne, France).

Antibiotic resistance of the identified Staphylococcal strains was determined using the disc diffusion method. Paper discs containing antibiotics were placed on Mueller-Hinton medium (BioMaxima, Lublin, Poland) inoculated with randomly selected strains of mannitol-positive staphylococci. Seven different groups of antibiotics of specified concentration (cefoxitin—FOX 30 µg; gentamycin—CN 10 µg; erythromycin—E 15 µg; tetracycline—TE 30 µg; chloramphenicol—C 30 µg; levofloxacin—LEV 5 µg; and rifampicin—RD 5 µg) were used to assess the full spectrum of resistance of the all strains. For *Staphylococcus aureus*, one more antibiotic—i.e., penicillin (P 1 unit)—was used in accordance with the guidelines of the European Committee on Antimicrobial Susceptibility Testing (EUCAST) [19]. After an 18-h incubation at 37 °C, we measured zones of inhibited growth formed around the discs. Subsequently, the investigated strains were divided into two groups: susceptible and resistant to antibiotics.

The concentration of molds was determined using Sabouraud's nutrient medium (BTL, Warszawa, Poland). These microorganisms were incubated at 26 °C for 5 days, after which time grown colonies were counted and their concentration was expressed as colony-forming units per cubic meter of air (CFU m^{-3}). For their identification, molds were transferred on Czapek-Dox medium and incubated at

26 °C for 5 days. Subsequently, microscope slides were prepared and stained with Shear's medium. Molds were identified on the basis of their macroscopic (colony diameter; colony color—reverse; colony structure; colony edge; colony center) and microscopic (vegetative mycelium, vegetative spores, chlamydospores) features according to Samson et al. [20].

2.3. Statistical Analysis

The Statistica 13.1 software was used for statistical analysis of the results. After log transformation, the results in the analyzed groups were normally distributed, which was confirmed using the Shapiro–Wilk test. In order to assess the impact of independent factors—i.e., time and place of sampling—on dependent variables—i.e., the concentrations of particular microbial groups—the ANOVA test was used. Tukey's multiple comparison analysis method (the posthoc Tukey's test) was conducted to compare the differences in the studied variables between the groups. In order to analyze relationships between the examined parameters, the Spearman correlation coefficient was determined. Statistical analyses were performed at the significance level of $p \leq 0.05$.

3. Results

In terms of surface area (size), libraries in both schools were the biggest studied rooms, followed by classrooms and cafeterias. The air temperature in School B was at a constant level—i.e., 22 °C—while in School A it was one degree higher in the classroom and the cafeteria than in the library (Table 1).

In both schools, the concentration of heterotrophic bacteria was correlated with the size of the studied rooms (Figure 1a,b). In rooms with a smaller surface area (the cafeterias), the concentration of heterotrophic bacteria was higher (School A: r = −0.63, $p = 0.005$; School B: r = −0.52, $p = 0.025$). A negative relationship was also observed for staphylococci (School A: r = −0.14; School B: r = −0.36), but the results were not statistically significant. On the other hand, the concentration of molds was not correlated with the size of the rooms in neither of the schools (r < 0.1, $p > 0.05$). The air temperature was similar in all the investigated rooms in School A and the same, in School B. (Table 1). Therefore, this factor did not significantly affect microbial concentration.

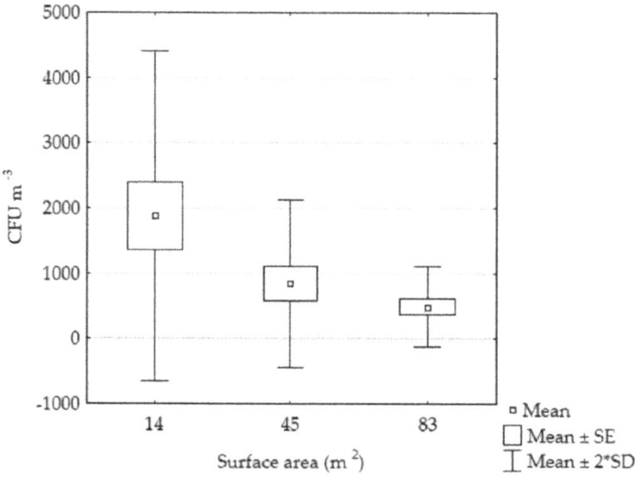

(a)

Figure 1. *Cont.*

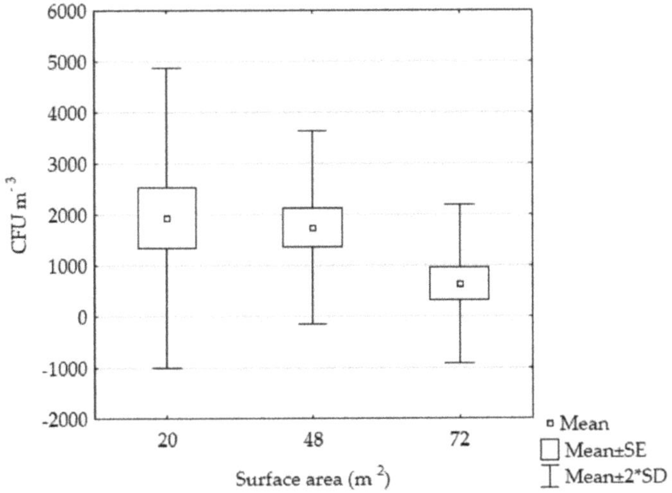

(**b**)

Figure 1. The relationship between (**a**) the size of the areas in School A and the total concentration of heterotrophic bacteria and (**b**) the size of the areas in School B and the total number of heterotrophic bacteria. SE—standard error; SD—standard deviation.

3.1. Concentrations of Bacterial Bioaerosol

In the air of the studied rooms, heterotrophic bacteria were the most abundant, and their concentrations ranged from 93 to 6070 CFU m^{-3} (Table 2).

Table 2. Number of heterotrophic bacteria in air (CFU m^{-3}).

Sampling Sites		Month of Sampling						M ± SD
		September	October	November	December	January	February	
School A	I—classroom	1607	1357	1266	546	219	93	848 ± 643
	II—library	430	480	1050	333	520	133	491 ± 307
	III—cafeteria	2120	3047	3593	1397	527	620	1884 ± 1265
M ± SD		1386 ± 866	1628 ± 1305	1970 ± 1410	759 ± 563	422 ± 176	282 ± 293	
School B	IV—classroom	347	1613	2776	2762	899	1949	1724 ± 982
	V—library	387	2143	190	393	160	150	571 ± 778
	VI—cafeteria	373	880	3077	4080	6070	2353	1906 ± 1499
M ± SD		625 ± 189	1545 ± 634	2014 ± 1587	2412 ± 1868	576 ± 378	1484 ± 1173	

M—mean; SD—standard deviation.

The highest average concentrations of airborne heterotrophic bacteria were recorded in the cafeterias—i.e., 1884 (School A) and 1906 CFU m^{-3} (School B)—and in the classrooms—i.e., 848 (School A) and 1724 CFU m^{-3} (School B). The lowest average concentration of airborne heterotrophic bacteria in the studied schools was noted in the libraries: 491 (School A) and 571 CFU m^{-3} (School B) (Table 2). In the present study, the concentration of heterotrophic bacteria increased in the period from November to February in the cafeteria in School B, with maximum values recorded in January. In November, December and February, relatively high concentrations of these bacteria were recorded in the classroom in the same school (Table 2).

There were statistically significant differences in the concentration of heterotrophic bacteria depending on the sampling sites in School A ($F = 4.47$, $p = 0.03$) and School B ($F = 4.59$, $p = 0.027$). The concentration of these microorganisms in School A was significantly higher in the cafeteria than in the library ($p = 0.029$). On the other hand, in School B, the concentration of heterotrophic bacteria in the class and cafeteria was statistically significantly higher than in the library, with $p = 0.046$ and $p = 0.049$, respectively. The concentration of heterotrophic bacteria was not correlated with the sampling month (Table 3).

Table 3. Statistical differences in microbial concentrations depending on a sampling site and sampling month.

	Microorganisms	F	*p*	Differences	F	*p*	Differences
	Sampling Sites				**Month of Sampling**		
School A	Heterotrophic bacteria	**4.47**	**0.030**	II:III *	1.74	0.2	ns
	Fungi	0.02	0.984	ns	**23.43**	**<0.001**	S:D **; S:J **; S:F *;O:D ***; O:J ***; O:F ***; N:D **, N:J **; N:F **
	Staphylococci	1.31	0.299	ns	1.57	0.242	ns
School B	Heterotrophic bacteria	**4.59**	**0.028**	V:IV *; VI:IV *	1.22	0.358	ns
	Fungi	0.12	0.889	ns	**13.66**	**<0.001**	S:D *; S:J **; S:F **; O:D *; O:J **; O:F **; N:J *
	Staphylococci	1.57	0.241	ns	1.59	0.236	ns

F—statistic ratio for ANOVA analysis; *p*—probability value. The bold *p* indicates a significant difference ($p < 0.05$) between the numbers of microorganisms in dependent of sampling sites (School A: I—classroom, II—library, III—cafeteria; School B: IV—classroom; V—library, VI—cafeteria) and month of sampling (September (S), October (O), November (N), December (D), January (J), February (F)). Differences—multiple comparisons (Tukey's HSD test); ns—differences statistically non-significant; *—$p \leq 0.05$; **—$p \leq 0.01$; ***—$p \leq 0.001$.

3.2. Concentrations of Fungal Bioaerosol

In the air of the studied schools, the concentration of molds ranged from 3 to 840 CFU m^{-3} (Table 4). The average concentrations of molds in all the investigated school rooms (classrooms, libraries, cafeterias) were similar and amounted to above 160 CFU m^{-3} in School A and around 300 CFU m^{-3} in School B (Table 4). There were no statistically significant correlations between mold levels and the sampling site.

Table 4. Number of fungi in air (CFU m^{-3}).

Sampling Sites		Month of Sampling						M ± SD
		September	October	November	December	January	February	
School A	I—classroom	283	297	230	30	13	113	161 ± 126
	II—library	220	460	290	40	3	37	175 ± 181
	III—cafeteria	263	283	270	80	27	107	172 ± 113
M ± SD		255 ± 32	347 ± 98	263 ± 31	50 ± 26	14 ± 12	86 ± 42	
School B	IV—classroom	487	457	380	297	37	97	293 ± 188
	V—library	840	690	310	57	37	117	342 ± 345
	VI—cafeteria	547	660	483	310	56	137	366 ± 239
M ± SD		625 ± 189	602 ± 127	391 ± 87	221 ± 142	43 ± 11	117 ± 20	

M—mean; SD—standard deviation.

In the present study, there were statistically significant differences in mold level depending on the sampling month ($p < 0.001$). In School A, average mold concentration was significantly higher ($p < 0.01$–$p < 0.001$) in autumn months—i.e., September, October and November—compared to December, January and February. A similar pattern was observed in School B: statistically significantly lower average mold concentrations ($p < 0.016$–$p < 0.001$) were also recorded in winter months—i.e., December, January and February—as compared to September and October. Mold concentration in November differed significantly ($p = 0.027$) only in relation to January (Table 3).

3.3. Predominant Genera of Airborne Fungi

In the investigated schools, *Cladosporium* prevailed in fungal bioaerosol at the majority of the sampling sites. Their highest concentrations were recorded in the libraries of both schools: School A (59%), School B (54%), in the classroom in School B (47%), and in the cafeteria in School A (50%).

Lower concentration—i.e., 35%—was noted in the classroom in School A and in the cafeteria in School B (Figure 2). The exception was the cafeteria in School B, dominated by *Penicillium* spores accounting for 42% of the fungal bioaerosol. They had a slightly smaller share in the cafeteria in School A (30%), in the classroom in School A (28%) and in the classroom in School B (22%). In the library in School A, *Penicillium* had a share of 12% and in the library in School B (10%) (Figure 2).

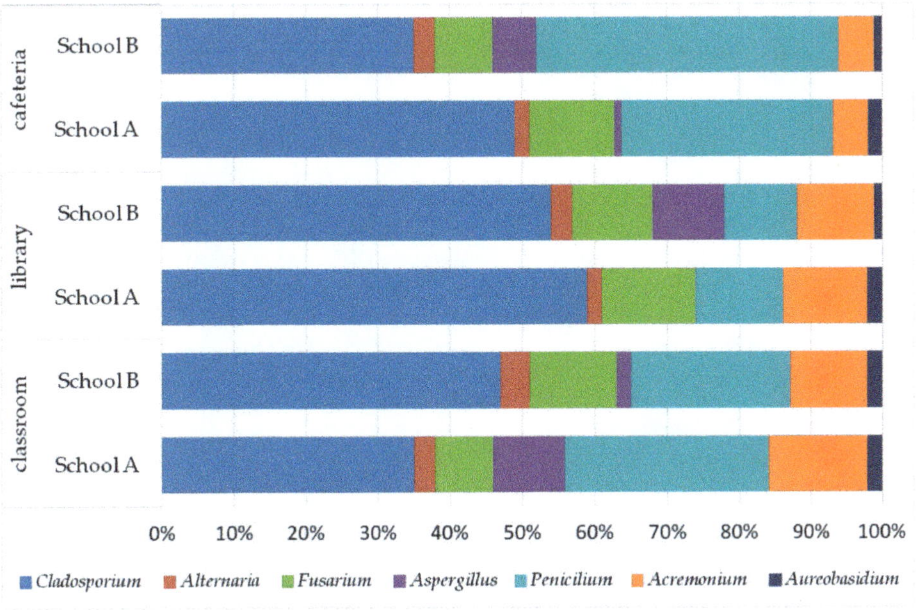

Figure 2. Predominant genera of airborne fungi at all sampling sites.

In the present study, *Fusarium* and *Acremonium* species were recorded alongside *Cladosporium* and *Penicillum*. At all sampling sites, they had a similar share in the fungal bioaerosol, ranging from 8 to 13% and 5 to 12%, respectively. *Aspergillus* spores were also identified, accounting for 10% of fungal bioaerosol in the classroom in School A and in the library in School B, and for 6% in the cafeteria in School B. They were not identified in the library in School A but constituted 1–2% of the fungal bioaerosol in the classroom in School B and in the cafeteria in School A. The spores of *Alternaria* and *Aureobasidium* constituted the lowest percentage of fungal bioaerosol in the studied school rooms (2–4% and 1–2%, respectively) (Figure 2).

3.4. Concentrations of Mannitol-Positive Staphylococci and Their Identification

In the studied schools, the concentration of staphylococci ranged from 0 to 16 CFU m^{-3}, with the maximum recorded in October in the cafeterias in both schools and the library in School B. No mannitol-positive staphylococci were recorded in September in the cafeteria, in November in the classroom in School B or in January in the classroom in School A (Table 5). There were no statistically significant differences in the concentration of staphylococci depending on the sampling site or sampling month (Table 3).

Table 5. Number of mannitol-positive staphylococci in air (CFU m^{-3}).

Sampling Sites		Month of Sampling						M ± SD
		September	October	November	December	January	February	
School A	I—classroom	10	13	10	3	0	6	7 ± 5
	II—library	6	10	3	6	3	10	6 ± 3
	III—cafeteria	3	16	13	6	13	10	10 ± 5
M ± SD		6 ± 3	13 ± 3	9 ± 5	5 ± 2	5 ± 7	9 ± 2	
School B	IV—classroom	3	10	0	10	13	3	7 ± 5
	V—library	13	16	3	13	6	6	10 ± 5
	VI—cafeteria	0	16	13	13	13	13	11 ± 6
M ± SD		5 ± 7	14 ± 3	5 ± 7	12 ± 2	11 ± 4	7 ± 5	

M—mean; SD—standard deviation.

In the air of the investigated schools in Bydgoszcz, *Staphylococcus aureus* was the dominant species, constituting 43% of all mannitol-positive staphylococci in School B and 26% in School A (Table 6). *Staphylococcus xylosus* (25%) and *Staphylococcus haemolyticus* (17%) had a slightly smaller share in the airborne staphylococcal population in School A, while each of the remaining 4 species—i.e., *S. cohnii* spp. *cohnii*, *S. chromogenes*, *S. lentus* and *S. saprophyticus*—accounted for only 4%. In School B, the species composition of mannitol-positive staphylococci was less diverse with four species identified apart from *S. aureus*: *S. saprophyticus* (25%), *S. xylosus* (16%), *S. haemolyticus* (8%) and *S. capities* (8%) (Table 6).

Table 6. Species diversity of the genus *Staphylococcus*.

Phylum	Class	Order	Family	Genus/Species	Percentage	
					School A	School B
Firmicutes	*Bacilli*	*Bacillales*	*Staphylococcaceae*	*Staphylococcus haemolyticus*	17%	8%
				Staphylococcus aureus	26%	43%
				Staphylococcus cohnii spp. *cohnii*	8%	0%
				Staphylococcus chromogenes	8%	0%
				Staphylococcus lentus	8%	0%
				Staphylococcus saprophyticus	8%	25%
				Staphylococcus xylosus	25%	16%
				Staphylococcus capities	0%	8%

3.5. Antimicrobial Resistance of Staphylococci

All isolated mannitol-positive staphylococcal strains (n = 24) were susceptible to levofloxacin and gentamicin (100%), while 62.5% were resistant to erythromycin. Some staphylococcal strains also showed resistance to tetracycline (20.8%) and cefoxitin (25%) (Table 7). Penicillin, which was used only for *Staphylococcus aureus*, turned out to be ineffective. All *Staphylococcus aureus* isolates (n = 8) showed resistance to this antibiotic.

Table 7. Antibiotic resistance of staphylococci, determined by the disc diffusion method.

No.	Species	Antibiotic Resistance							
		P1	E15	RD5	CN10	FOX30	TE30	C30	LEV5
1.	*S. saprophyticus*		R	-	-	-	-	-	-
2.	*S. saprophyticus*		R	-	-	-	-	-	-
3.	*S. saprophyticus*		R	-	-	-	-	R	-
4.	*S. saprophyticus*		R	-	-	-	-	-	-
5.	*S. xylosus*		R	-	-	-	-	-	-
6.	*S. xylosus*		-	-	-	-	-	-	-
7.	*S. xylosus*		R	-	-	-	-	-	-

Table 7. *Cont.*

No.	Species	Antibiotic Resistance							
		P1	E15	RD5	CN10	FOX30	TE30	C30	LEV5
8.	*S. xylosus*		R	-	-	-	-	-	-
9.	*S.xylosus*		R	-	-	-	-	-	-
10.	*S. haemolyticus*		-	-	-	R	-	-	-
11.	*S. haemolyticus*		-	-	-	R	-	-	-
12.	*S. haemolyticus*		R	-	-	R	-	-	-
13.	*S. aureus*	R	-	-	-	-	R	-	-
14.	*S. aureus*	R	-	-	-	-	R	-	-
15.	*S. aureus*	R	-	-	-	-	R	-	-
16.	*S. aureus*	R	R	-	-	-	-	-	-
17.	*S. aureus*	R	R	-	-	-	-	-	-
18.	*S. aureus*	R	-	-	-	R	R	-	-
19.	*S. aureus*	R	-	-	-	-	-	-	-
20.	*S. aureus*	R	-	-	-	-	R	-	-
21.	*S.cohnii* spp. *cohnii*		R	-	-	R	-	R	-
22.	*S. chromogenes*		R	-	-	-	-	-	-
23.	*S. lentus*		R	R	-	R	-	-	-
24.	*S. capitis*		R	-	-	-	-	-	-
Percent of resistance		100%	62.5%	4.2%	0%	25.0%	20.8%	8.3%	0%

(R)—resistant; (-)—susceptible; P1—benzylpenicillin; E15—erythromycin; RD5—rifampicin; CN10—gentamicin; FOX30—cefoxitin; TE30—tetracycline; C30—chloramphenicol; LEV5—levofloxacin.

4. Discussion

Bioaerosols are always present in the air and contain contaminant particles including pollen and microorganisms such as bacteria, fungi and viruses [21,22]. As indicators of air quality, they play a key role in air quality and health risk assessment [23–27]. They can reduce air quality in educational institutions [11,28]. According to Brągoszewska [25], indoor air is often polluted by microbial bioaerosols, which are, therefore, a major public health concern.

4.1. Bacterial Bioaresol Concentration

The results presented in the previous section (Section 3.1) indicated that heterotrophic bacteria were the most numerous microorganisms and that their concentrations were similar to those reported by other authors. Madureira [29] in Porto, Portugal recorded a minimum of 268 CFU m^{-3} and a maximum of 8512 CFU m^{-3}, while Andualem et al. [5] in Gondar city, Ethiopia, recorded concentrations ranging from 208 to 9100 CFU m^{-3} in the morning but much higher, ranging from 260 to 23,504 CFU m^{-3} in the afternoon. Slightly lower maximum levels of heterotrophic bacteria were noted by Brągoszewska et al. [3] in rural nursery schools in the Upper Silesia region of Poland (2600 CFU m^{-3}) and by Mainka et al. [30] and Brągoszewska et al. [22] in a nursery school in Gliwice, Poland—i.e., over 3000 CFU m^{-3}. In the studied schools, the highest average concentrations of heterotrophic bacteria were recorded in the cafeterias and classrooms, which tend to be occupied by higher numbers of students and for longer periods of time than libraries. High average concentrations of these microorganisms in these rooms were similar to those reported by Brągoszewska et al. [13] in the primary school (2205 CFU m^{-3}) and nursery school (1408 CFU m^{-3}) in the industrial region of Upper Silesia, Poland. These results differ significantly from those obtained by other researchers, who recorded lower numbers of these microorganisms. In the study by Madureira et al. [31], an average bacterial concentration in schools in Porto, Portugal was 332 CFU m^{-3}. Similar levels were noted by Yang et al. [32] in schools in Seoul, Korea, where the average concentration of heterotrophic bacteria was 451 CFU m^{-3} in the classroom and 297 CFU m^{-3} in the laboratory. Air quality research conducted by Sheik et al. [33] in Saudi Arabia showed a similar average concentration of bacterial bioaerosol in classrooms—i.e., 290 CFU m^{-3}. Much lower average concentrations of heterotrophic bacteria—i.e.,

87 CFU m^{-3}—were recorded by Kallawicha et al. [34] in laboratories in Bangkok, Thailand, which can be associated with different climate, type of ventilation, number of users and their activities. Brągoszewska and Biedroń [11] emphasize the importance of adequate ventilation for microbiological air quality. The researchers recorded the highest average concentrations of heterotrophic bacteria in school offices in Gliwice, Poland in April (821 CFU m^{-3}), when the rooms were not aired regularly and the lowest, in June (424 CFU m^{-3}), when the rooms were well-aired.

Furthermore, as stated by Dumała and Dzudzińska [35] and Al Mijalli [36], microbiological air contamination in school rooms depends on many factors, the most important being the number of children and their physical activity.

According to Fang et al. [37], bacterial concentration in the air is also influenced by meteorological and environmental conditions. Brągoszewska and Pastuszka [22] report that it depends on the geographical location of the investigated facility and seasonal variations in the bacterial community structure. Mentese et al. [38] emphasize that in Ankara, Turkey, the highest microbial concentrations were observed in nursery schools—i.e., 649 CFU m^{-3} in winter and 1462 CFU m^{-3} in summer. Wolny-Kołladka et al. [1] noted that in November, the critical values for bacteria were exceeded in an university office, toilet and corridor, and in June and September, in the biomass analysis laboratory.

4.2. Concentrations of Fungal Bioaerosol

Mold level in indoor air is associated with many factors: outdoor air pollutants, room ventilation, building materials, building maintenance, number of occupants in the room and mold infestation of the building [29,39,40]. Poor air quality may lead to lung diseases and allergies and cause non-specific symptoms known as sick building syndrome [41].

In the air of the studied schools, the concentration of molds was much lower than that of heterotrophic bacteria. Similar results were obtained by Kalwasińska et al. [42] examining air quality in the university library in Toruń, Poland. Comparable ranges were also noted by Brągoszewska et al. [3] in rural nursery schools in the Upper Silesia region of Poland (78–788 CFU m^{-3}). In Portuguese primary schools, a higher concentration range—i.e., 16–1792 CFU m^{-3}—was reported by Madureira et al. [31]. However, in nursery schools in Ankara, Turkey, lower levels of fungal aerosols—i.e., 27–53 CFU m^{-3}—were observed by Mentese et al. [43]. In our study, the average concentrations of molds in all the investigated rooms in School B were higher and amounted to approximately 300 CFU m^{-3}. Many researchers have recorded similar average values—i.e., 332 [31] and 368 CFU m^{-3} in school rooms [3] and 294.9 CFU m^{-3} in laboratories [34]. Mold level was lower at all sampling sites in winter, which is consistent with literature reports. Wolny-Kołladka et al. [1] also recorded lower concentrations of molds at the University of Agriculture in Cracow in winter compared to other seasons.

4.3. Predominant Genera of Airborne Fungi

The presence of mold spores in indoor air is very common because they can survive on furniture, equipment, in ventilation systems, etc. for a long time [44]. Many mold species are associated with allergic reactions including respiratory and skin symptoms, mainly in people with immunodeficiency [45]. The most clinically important allergens are produced by fungi belonging to the following genera: *Alternaria, Aspergillus, Cladosporium, Mucor, Penicilium* and *Fusarium* [46,47].

Cladosporium species, ubiquitous worldwide, represent the most frequently isolated airborne fungi, especially in the temperate zone [48–50]. This observation is consistent with our results.

In studies by Madureira et al. [51] fungal bioaerosol in primary schools and childcare centers was dominated by *Penicillium* and *Cladosporium* species. Viegas et al. [52] recorded a variety of molds in gyms with swimming pools, with the highest shares of *Cladosporium* sp. (36.6%), *Penicillium* (19%), *Aspergillus* sp. (10.2%) and *Mucor* (7%).

Kallawich et al. [34] observed that *Aspergillus/Penicillium* were the most abundant fungal taxa in the laboratories (40.6%), followed by *Cladosporium* (30%) and ascospores (17%). Similarly, Verde et al. [53] confirmed the dominance of *Penicillium* (41%) and *Aspergillus* (24%) in the air of hospital rooms.

According to Cabral [54], high humidity in sick buildings promotes fungal growth (mainly of *Penicillium* and *Aspergillus* species) with the release of conidia and cell fragments into the atmosphere.

4.4. Concentrations of Mannitol-Positive Staphylococci and Their Identification

Staphylococci are abundant bacteria of the human skin microbiome [55] that often do not cause infections. However, in certain circumstances, they may pose a threat to both immunocompetent people and people whose immune system is weakened or impaired [1].

Manniotol-positive staphylococci were identified in the air of the studied schools in Bydgoszcz, but their concentrations were lower than those reported by Wolny-Koładka et al. [1] at the university—i.e., from 0 to 65 CFU m^{-3}. According to Boada et al. [56], one fifth of the population (mainly children) are persistent carriers of *S. aureus* This seems to have been confirmed by our results, which indicated that this particular species dominated among the identified staphylococci. The species composition of airborne staphylococci in Bydgoszcz schools was similar to that in the University of Ibadan library in Nigeria [57] where *S. aureus*, *S. arlattae*, *S. cohnii*, *S. haemolyticus* and *S. muscae* were identified. Different results were obtained by Wolny-Koładka et al. [1] at the University of Agricultural in Cracow, where three dominant species—i.e., *S. xylosus* (18%), *S. sciuri* (17%) and *S. hominis* (15%)—were distinguished. At the same time, Brągoszewska et al. [13] identified four staphylococcal species in three educational buildings in the industrial region of Upper Silesia, Poland, namely *S. lentus*, *S. epidermidis*, *S. sciuri* and *S. chromogenes*, while Brągoszewska et al. [58] confirmed the dominance of *S. lentus*, *S. epidermidis* and *S. chromogens* in the high school gym located in an urban area of Southern Poland.

4.5. Antimicrobial Resistance of Staphylococci

The presence of airborne *Staphylococcus* spp. indicates the possible presence of pathogenic microorganisms, in which antibiotic resistance has been observed with increasing frequency over the past several decades. According to Peterson et al. [59], the growth of antibiotic-resistant bacteria poses a serious threat to public health, food security and development today. The importance of this problem on a global scale is emphasized by the World Health Organization [60], which warns that without urgent action, the world is heading for a post-antibiotic era. Moreover, WHO indicates that when new resistance mechanisms are emerging and spreading globally, there is increased demand for new drugs, while the possibilities of obtaining them are currently very limited.

Antibiotic resistance is associated mainly with overuse and misuse of these medications [61,62]. Bacterial strains acquire resistance which spreads rapidly even to modern drugs [63]. Among the factors contributing to the emergence of drug resistance is bacterial ability to adapt to environmental conditions through biofilm formation, which facilitates the spread of their resistance genes [64]. In order to survive stress triggered by antibiotics, bacteria alter their gene expression and activate latent defense mechanisms [65]. A shortage of new drugs and the availability of non-prescription antibiotics combined with the rapid growth of multidrug-resistance in bacteria necessitate an interdisciplinary approach to complementary and alternative treatments [66,67].

The analysis conducted in two Bydgoszcz schools indicated both resistance and sensitivity to selected antibiotics in the isolated Staphyloccocal strains. Levofloxacin and gentamicin turned out to be the most effective medicines. Similar results were obtained by Małecka-Adamowicz et al. [68] investigating the antibiotic resistance of staphylococci isolated from the air in several sports facilities in Bydgoszcz. Sensitivity to levofloxacin most likely results from its increased activity against Gram-positive microorganisms [69]. In the present study the isolated staphylococci had the highest resistance to erythromycin (62.5%). Comparable results were obtained by Frías-De León et al. [70] and Lenart-Boroń et al. [62].

In the study by Wolny-Koładka et al. [1], more than 50% of staphylococci isolated from the air on the premises of the University of Agricultural in Cracow were resistant to erythromycin and about 33%, to tetracycline. A much higher resistance to tetracycline (75% of strains) was recorded by Giwa et al. [57] in the air of university libraries in Ibadan, Nigeria. According to Lenart-Boroń et al. [71], high resistance of the studied strains to erythromycin and tetracycline may stem from the fact that these antibiotics have been in use for a long time, which may have contributed to the increased resistance of bacteria to these drugs.

As recommended by the European Committee for Susceptibility Testing [19], the analysis of susceptibility to penicillin was performed only for *S. aureus* due to fact that no currently available method can reliably detect penicillinase production in coagulase-negative staphylococci. All isolated *S. aureus* strains were penicillin resistant, which is connected with their ability to produce penicillinase. More than 90% of all staphylococci are capable of producing this enzyme, resulting in their resistance to most penicillins [19].

The rapid emergence of resistant bacteria, which occurs worldwide, endangers the efficacy of antibiotics and may lead to a serious crisis in healthcare. Therefore, a need for better understanding of antibiotic-resistant bacterial populations is obvious [23]. In view of that, the monitoring of air quality in schools in order to assess bacterial acquisition of antibiotic resistance seems a necessary measure.

Exposure to bioaerosols has become a serious health problem. However, no international standards specifying its acceptable maximum levels for indoor environments are available [72].

In addition, it should be emphasized that with the use of different equipment and sampling methods it is not possible to provide a reliable comparison of the results obtained by different researchers [73]. Therefore, relevant organizations should develop clear criteria for assessing indoor and outdoor air quality Wolny-Koładka et al. [1].

5. Conclusions

Our study was conducted in two schools in northern Poland, where air samples were collected not only from classrooms (standard approach) but also from libraries and cafeterias, which are frequently used by students. The results led to the following conclusions:

1. A statistically significant relationship between the size of the rooms and the concentration of heterotrophic bacteria was observed. In both schools, higher microbial concentrations were recorded in smaller rooms (the cafeterias). There were no statistically significant differences in the concentration of molds and staphylococci depending on the sampling site. The average concentrations of these groups of microorganisms was similar in the studied rooms.
2. In both schools, only mold concentration significantly depended on the sampling month ($p < 0.001$), which may be connected with relative humidity.
3. The air temperature was similar in all the investigated rooms; therefore, this factor did not significantly affect microbial concentration.
4. In the air of the investigated school rooms, *Cladosporium* and *Penicillium* species were dominant fungi, which may be related to the use of natural ventilation—i.e., opening the windows—allowing the inflow of these molds from the outside.
5. The taxonomic analysis indicated that *Staphylococcus aureus* dominated among mannitol-positive staphylococci in both schools, while *S. xylosus*, *S. haemolyticus* and *S. saprophyticus* were slightly less abundant. The predominance of the opportunistic *Staphylococcus aureus* in the air of the studied schools confirms the observation that there are carriers of this bacteria among students.
6. Antibiogram patterns of the isolated staphylococcal strains showed their high resistance to erythromycin, while levofloxacin and gentamicin were the most effective antibiotics. No spread of multidrug-resistant staphylococcal strains in the air of the studied schools was observed.

Our research may serve as a basis for future studies, which should be supplemented with measurements of particulate matter (PM) (with special emphasis on respirable PM) and of physicochemical parameters. The amount of aerosol inhaled by room users should also be determined. In addition, given the current lack of precise indoor air quality guidelines in Poland, the research may be a valuable contribution.

Author Contributions: Conceptualization, M.M.-A.; Data curation, M.M.-A.; Methodology, M.M.-A. and B.K.-P.; Supervision, M.M.-A.; Visualization, M.M.-A.; Writing—original draft, M.M.-A., B.K.-P. and E.A.D.; Writing—review and editing, M.M.-A., B.K.-P. and E.A.D. All authors have read and agreed to the published version of the manuscript.

Funding: This paper was funded by the Polish Minister of Science and Higher Education under the programme "Regional Initiative of Excellence" in 2019–2022 (Grant No. 008/RID/2018/19).

Conflicts of Interest: The authors declare no conflict of interest.

References

1. Wolny-Kołladka, K.; Malinowski, M.; Pieklik, A.; Kurpaska, S. Microbiological air contamination in university premises and the evaluation of drug resistance of staphylococci occurring in the form of a bioaerosol. *Indoor Built Environ.* **2017**, *28*, 235–246. [CrossRef]
2. Meadow, J.F.; Altrichter, A.E.; Kembel, S.W.; Kline, J.; Mhuireach, G.; Moriyama, M.; Northcutt, D.; O'Connor, T.K.; Womack, A.M.; Brown, G.Z.; et al. Indoor airborne bacterial communities are influenced by ventilation, occupancy, and outdoor air source. *Indoor Air* **2013**, *24*, 41–48. [CrossRef]
3. Brągoszewska, E.; Mainka, A.; Pastuszka, J.S. Bacterial and Fungal Aerosols in Rural Nursery Schools in Southern Poland. *Atmosphere* **2016**, *7*, 142. [CrossRef]
4. Ramos, C.; Wolterbeek, H.; Almeida, S. Exposure to indoor air pollutants during physical activity in fitness centers. *Build. Environ.* **2014**, *82*, 349–360. [CrossRef]
5. Andualem, Z.; Gizaw, Z.; Bogale, L.; Dagne, H. Indoor bacterial load and its correlation to physical indoor air quality parameters in public primary schools. *Multidiscip. Respir. Med.* **2019**, *14*, 2. [CrossRef]
6. Naruka, K.; Gaur, J. Microbial air contamination in a school. *Int. J. Curr. Microbiol. App. Sci.* **2013**, *2*, 404–405.
7. Canha, N.; Almeida, S.; Freitas, M.C.; Täubel, M.; Hänninen, O. Winter Ventilation Rates at Primary Schools: Comparison between Portugal and Finland. *J. Toxicol. Environ. Health Part A* **2013**, *76*, 400–408. [CrossRef]
8. Patelarou, E.; Tzanakis, N.; Kelly, F.J. Exposure to Indoor Pollutants and Wheeze and Asthma Development during Early Childhood. *Int. J. Environ. Res. Public Health* **2015**, *12*, 3993–4017. [CrossRef]
9. Mainka, A.; Zajusz-Zubek, E. Indoor Air Quality in Urban and Rural Preschools in Upper Silesia, Poland: Particulate Matter and Carbon Dioxide. *Int. J. Environ. Res. Public Health* **2015**, *12*, 7697–7711. [CrossRef] [PubMed]
10. Du, P.; Du, R.; Lu, Z.; Ren, W.; Fu, P. Variation of Bacterial and Fungal Community Structures in PM2.5 Collected during the 2014 APEC Summit Periods. *Aerosol Air Qual. Res.* **2018**, *18*, 444–455. [CrossRef]
11. Brągoszewska, E.; Biedroń, I.; Kozielska, B.; Pastuszka, J.S. Microbiological indoor air quality in an office building in Gliwice, Poland: Analysis of the case study. *Air Qual. Atmos. Health* **2018**, *11*, 729–740. [CrossRef]
12. Fsadni, P.; Frank, B.; Fsadni, C.; Montefort, S. The Impact of Microbiological Pollutants on School Indoor Air Quality. *J. Geosci. Environ. Prot.* **2017**, *5*, 54–65. [CrossRef]
13. Brągoszewska, E.; Mainka, A.; Pastuszka, J.S.; Lizończyk, K.; Desta, Y.G. Assessment of Bacterial Aerosol in a Preschool, Primary School and High School in Poland. *Atmosphere* **2018**, *9*, 87. [CrossRef]
14. Demirel, G.; Özden, Ö; Döğeroğlu, T.; Gaga, E.O. Personal exposure of primary school children to BTEX, NO_2 and ozone in Eskişehir, Turkey: Relationship with indoor/outdoor concentrations and risk assessment. *Sci. Total Environ.* **2014**, *473*, 537–548. [CrossRef]
15. Yoon, C.; Lee, K.; Park, N. Indoor air quality differences between urban and rural preschools in Korea. *Environ. Sci. Pollut. Res.* **2010**, *18*, 333–345. [CrossRef]
16. Labi, A.-K.; Obeng-Nkrumah, N.; Bjerrum, S.; Aryee, N.A.A.; Ofori-Adjei, Y.A.; Yawson, A.E.; Newman, M.J. Physicians' knowledge, attitudes, and perceptions concerning antibiotic resistance: A survey in a Ghanaian tertiary care hospital. *BMC Health Serv. Res.* **2018**, *18*, 126. [CrossRef]
17. Blaga, A.B. The importance of indoor air quality study in schools. *AMT* **2016**, *21*, 19.

18. Feller, W. *An Introduction to the Probability Theory and Its Application*; John Wiley & Sons Inc.: New York, NY, USA, 1950.
19. European Committee on Antimicrobial Susceptibility Testing—EUCAST. Breakpoint Tables for Interpretation of MICs and Zone Diameters. Version 8.1 2018. 2018. Available online: http://www.eucast.org (accessed on 15 May 2018).
20. Samson, R.A.; Hoekstra, E.S.; Frisvad, J.C. *Introduction to Food and Airborne Fungi*, 7th ed.; Centraalbureau voor Schimmelcultures: Utrecht, The Netherlands, 2004.
21. Tolabi, Z.; Alimohammadi, M.; Hassanvand, M.S.; Nabizadeh, R.; Soleimani, H.; Zarei, A. The investigation of type and concentration of bio-aerosols in the air of surgical rooms: A case study in Shariati hospital, Karaj. *MethodsX* **2019**, *6*, 641–650. [CrossRef] [PubMed]
22. Brągoszewska, E.; Pastuszka, J.S. Influence of meteorological factors on the level and characteristics of culturable bacteria in the air in Gliwice, Upper Silesia (Poland). *Aerobiology* **2018**, *34*, 241–255. [CrossRef] [PubMed]
23. Brągoszewska, E.; Biedroń, I.; Hryb, W. Microbiological Air Quality and Drug Resistance in Airborne Bacteria Isolated from a Waste Sorting Plant Located in Poland—A Case Study. *Microorganism* **2020**, *8*, 202. [CrossRef]
24. Jiayu, C.; Qiaoqiao, R.; Feilong, C.; Chen, L.; Jiguo, W.; Zhendong, W.; Lingyun, C.; Liu, R.; Guoxia, Z. Microbiology Community Structure in Bioaerosols and the Respiratory Diseases. *J. Environ. Sci. Public Health* **2019**, *3*, 347–357. [CrossRef]
25. Brągoszewska, E.; Bogacka, M.; Pikoń, K. Efficiency and Eco-Costs of Air Purifiers in Terms of Improving Microbiological Indoor Air Quality in Dwellings—A Case Study. *Atmosphere* **2019**, *10*, 742. [CrossRef]
26. Moore, M.N. Do airborne biogenic chemicals interact with the PI3K/Akt/mTOR cell signalling pathway to benefit human health and wellbeing in rural and coastal environments? *Environ. Res.* **2015**, *140*, 65–75. [CrossRef]
27. Cincinelli, A.; Martellini, T. Indoor Air Quality and Health. *Int. J. Environ. Res. Public Health* **2017**, *14*, 1286. [CrossRef] [PubMed]
28. Gizaw, Z.; Gebrehiwot, M.; Yenew, C. High bacterial load of indoor air in hospital wards: The case of University of Gondar teaching hospital, Northwest Ethiopia. *Multidiscip. Respir. Med.* **2016**, *11*, 24. [CrossRef] [PubMed]
29. Madureira, J.; Aguiar, L.; Pereira, C.C.; Mendes, A.; Querido, M.; Neves, P.; Teixeira, J.P. Indoor exposure to bioaerosol particles: Levels and implications for inhalation dose rates in schoolchildren. *Air Qual. Atmos. Health* **2018**, *11*, 955–964. [CrossRef]
30. Mainka, A.; Brągoszewska, E.; Kozielska, B.; Pastuszka, J.S.; Zajusz-Zubek, E. Indoor air quality in urban nursery schools in Gliwice, Poland: Analysis of the case study. *Atmos. Pollut. Res.* **2015**, *6*, 1098–1104. [CrossRef]
31. Madureira, J.; Paciência, I.; Fernandes, E.D.O. Levels and Indoor–Outdoor Relationships of Size-Specific Particulate Matter in Naturally Ventilated Portuguese Schools. *J. Toxicol. Environ. Health Part A* **2012**, *75*, 1423–1436. [CrossRef]
32. Yang, J.; Nam, I.; Yun, H.; Kim, J.; Oh, H.-J.; Lee, D.; Jeon, S.-M.; Yoo, S.-H.; Sohn, J.-R. Characteristics of indoor air quality at urban elementary schools in Seoul, Korea: Assessment of effect of surrounding environments. *Atmos. Pollut. Res.* **2015**, *6*, 1113–1122. [CrossRef]
33. Sheik, G.B.; Ismail, A.; Abd, A.; Rheam, A.; Saad, Z.; Shehri, A.; Bin, O.; Al, M. Assessment of Bacteria and Fungi in air from College of Applied Medical Sciences (Male) at AD-Dawadmi, Saudi Arabia. *Int. J. Sci. Technol. Res.* **2015**, *4*, 48–53.
34. Kallawicha, K.; Chao, H.J.; Kotchasatan, N. Bioaerosol levels and the indoor air quality of laboratories in Bangkok metropolis. *Aerobiologia* **2018**, *35*, 1–14. [CrossRef]
35. Dumała, S.M.; Dudzińska, M.R. Microbiological indoor air quality in Polish schools. *Annu. Set Environ. Prot.* **2013**, *15*, 231–244.
36. Al-Mijalli, S.H.S. Bacterial Contamination of Indoor Air in Schools of Riyadh, Saudi Arabia. *Air Water Borne Dis.* **2017**, *6*, 1–8. [CrossRef]
37. Fang, Z.; Guo, W.; Zhang, J.; Lou, X. Influence of Heat Events on the Composition of Airborne Bacterial Communities in Urban Ecosystems. *Int. J. Environ. Res. Public Health* **2018**, *15*, 2295. [CrossRef]
38. Mentese, S.; Rad, A.Y.; Arısoy, M.; Güllü, G. Seasonal and Spatial Variations of Bioaerosols in Indoor Urban Environments, Ankara, Turkey. *Indoor Built Environ.* **2011**, *21*, 797–810. [CrossRef]

39. Womack, A.M.; Bohannan, B.J.M.; Green, J.L. Biodiversity and biogeography of the atmosphere. *Philos. Trans. R. Soc. B Biol. Sci.* **2010**, *365*, 3645–3653. [CrossRef]
40. Bowers, R.M.; McCubbin, I.B.; Hallar, A.G.; Fierer, N. Seasonal variability in airborne bacterial communities at a high-elevation site. *Atmos. Environ.* **2012**, *50*, 41–49. [CrossRef]
41. Pallabi, P. Review on Common Microbiological Contamination Found in Hospital Air. *J. Microbiol. Pathol.* **2018**, *2*, 103.
42. Kalwasińska, A.; Burkowska, A.; Wilk, I. Microbial air contamination in indoor environment of a university library. *Ann. Agric. Environ. Med.* **2012**, *19*, 25–29.
43. Mentese, S.; Arısoy, M.; Rad, A.Y.; Güllü, G.; Arisoy, M. Bacteria and Fungi Levels in Various Indoor and Outdoor Environments in Ankara, Turkey. *Clean Soil Air Water* **2009**, *37*, 487–493. [CrossRef]
44. Kobza, J.; Pastuszka, J.S.; Brągoszewska, E. Do exposures to aerosols pose a risk to dental professionals? *Occup. Med.* **2018**, *68*, 454–458. [CrossRef]
45. Twaroch, T.E.; Curin, M.; Valenta, R.; Swoboda, I. Mold Allergens in Respiratory Allergy: From Structure to Therapy. *Allergy Asthma Immunol. Res.* **2015**, *7*, 205–220. [CrossRef] [PubMed]
46. Crameri, R.; Garbani, M.; Rhyner, C.; Huitema, C. Fungi: The neglected allergenic sources. *Allergy* **2013**, *69*, 176–185. [CrossRef] [PubMed]
47. Pusz, W.; Kita, W.; Weber, R. Microhabitat Influences the Occurrence of Airborne Fungi in Copper Mine in Poland. *J. Cave Karst Stud.* **2014**, *76*, 14–19. [CrossRef]
48. Almaguer, M.; Aira, M.J.; Rodríguez-Rajo, F.J.; Fernández-González, M.; Rojas-Flores, T.I. Thirty-four identifiable airborne fungal spores in Havana, Cuba. *Ann. Agric. Environ. Med.* **2015**, *22*, 215–220. [CrossRef]
49. Khan, M.; Perveen, A.; Qaiser, M. Seasonal and diurnal variation of atmospheric fungal spore concentrations in Hyderabad, Tandojam-Sindh and the effects of climatic conditions. *Pak. J. Bot.* **2016**, *48*, 1657–1663.
50. Antón, S.F.; De La Cruz, D.R.; Sánchez, J.S.; Reyes, E.S. Analysis of the airborne fungal spores present in the atmosphere of Salamanca (MW Spain): A preliminary survey. *Aerobiologia* **2019**, *35*, 447–462. [CrossRef]
51. Madureira, J.; Paciência, I.; Rufo, J.C.; Pereira, C.; Teixeira, J.P.; Fernandes, E.D.O. Assessment and determinants of airborne bacterial and fungal concentrations in different indoor environments: Homes, child day-care centres, primary schools and elderly care centres. *Atmos. Environ.* **2015**, *109*, 139–146. [CrossRef]
52. Viegas, C.; Alves, C.; Carolino, E.; Rosado, L.; Santos, C.S. Prevalence of Fungi in Indoor Air with Reference to Gymnasiums with Swimming Pools. *Indoor Built Environ.* **2010**, *19*, 555–561. [CrossRef]
53. Verde, S.C.; Almeida, S.; Matos, J.; Guerreiro, D.; Meneses, M.; Faria, T.; Botelho, D.; Santos, M.; Viegas, C. Microbiological assessment of indoor air quality at different hospital sites. *Res. Microbiol.* **2015**, *166*, 557–563. [CrossRef]
54. Cabral, J.P.S. Can we use indoor fungi as bioindicators of indoor air quality? Historical perspectives and open questions. *Sci. Total Environ.* **2010**, *408*, 4285–4295. [CrossRef]
55. Tršan, M.; Seme, K.; Srčič, S. The environmental monitoring in hospital pharmacy cleanroom and microbiota catalogue preparation. *Saudi Pharm. J.* **2019**, *27*, 455–462. [CrossRef] [PubMed]
56. Boada, A.; Pons-Vigués, M.; Real, J.; Grezner, E.; Bolíbar, B.; Llor, C. Previous antibiotic exposure and antibiotic resistance of commensal *Staphylococcus aureus* in Spanish primary care. *Eur. J. Gen. Pract.* **2018**, *24*, 125–130. [CrossRef]
57. Giwa, H.J.; Ogunjobi, A.A. Prevalence of multiple antibiotic resistant bacteria in selected libraries of University of Ibadan, Nigeria. *J. Am. Sci.* **2017**, *13*, 18–25. [CrossRef]
58. Brągoszewska, E.; Biedroń, I.; Mainka, A. Microbiological Air Quality in a Highschool Gym Located in an Urban Area of Southern Poland—Preliminary Research. *Atmosphere* **2020**, *11*, 797. [CrossRef]
59. Peterson, E.; Kaur, P. Antibiotic Resistance Mechanisms in Bacteria: Relationships Between Resistance Determinants of Antibiotic Producers, Environmental Bacteria, and Clinical Pathogens. *Front. Microbiol.* **2018**, *9*, 2928. [CrossRef]
60. WHO—World Health Organization. *Antimicrobial Resistance Global Report on Surveillance*; World Health Organizations: Geneva, Switzerland, 2014.
61. Alhomoud, F.; Almahasnah, R.; Alhomoud, F.K. "You could lose when you misuse"—Factors affecting over-the-counter sale of antibiotics in community pharmacies in Saudi Arabia: A qualitative study. *BMC Health Serv. Res.* **2018**, *18*, 915. [CrossRef]

62. Lenart-Boron, A.; Wolny-Koładka, K.; Juraszek, K.; Kasprowicz, A. Phenotypic and molecular assessment of antimicrobial resistance profile of airborne *Staphylococcus* spp. isolated from flats in Kraków. *Aerobiologia* **2017**, *33*, 435–444. [CrossRef] [PubMed]
63. Nahaei, M.R.; Shahmohammadi, M.R.; Ebrahimi, S.; Milani, M. Detection of Methicillin-Resistant Coagulase-Negative Staphylococci and Surveillance of Antibacterial Resistance in a Multi-Center Study from Iran. *Jundishapur J. Microbiol.* **2015**, *8*, e19945. [CrossRef]
64. Brągoszewska, E.; Biedroń, I. Indoor Air Quality and Potential Health Risk Impacts of Exposure to Antibiotic Resistant Bacteria in an Office Rooms in Southern Poland. *Int. J. Environ. Res. Public Health* **2018**, *15*, 2604. [CrossRef]
65. Palmer, A.; Chait, R.; Kishony, R. Nonoptimal Gene Expression Creates Latent Potential for Antibiotic Resistance. *Mol. Biol. Evol.* **2018**, *35*, 2669–2684. [CrossRef] [PubMed]
66. Aslam, B.; Wang, W.; Arshad, M.I.; Khurshid, M.; Muzammil, S.; Rasool, M.H.; Nisar, M.A.; Alvi, R.F.; Aslam, M.A.; Qamar, M.U.; et al. Antibiotic resistance: A rundown of a global crisis. *Infect. Drug Resist.* **2018**, *11*, 1645–1658. [CrossRef] [PubMed]
67. Horumpende, P.G.; Sonda, T.B.; Van Zwetselaar, M.; Antony, M.L.; Tenu, F.F.; Mwanziva, C.E.; Shao, E.R.; Mshana, S.E.; Mmbaga, B.T.; Chilongola, J.O. Prescription and non-prescription antibiotic dispensing practices in part I and part II pharmacies in Moshi Municipality, Kilimanjaro Region in Tanzania: A simulated clients approach. *PLoS ONE* **2018**, *13*, e0207465. [CrossRef]
68. Małecka-Adamowicz, M.; Kubera, Ł.; Jankowiak, E.; Dembowska, E. Microbial diversity of bioaerosol inside sports facilities and antibiotic resistance of isolated *Staphylococcus* spp. *Aerobiologia* **2019**, *35*, 731–742. [CrossRef]
69. May, L.; Klein, E.Y.; Rothman, R.E.; Laxminarayan, R. Trends in Antibiotic Resistance in Coagulase-Negative Staphylococci in the United States, 1999 to 2012. *Antimicrob. Agents Chemother.* **2013**, *58*, 1404–1409. [CrossRef]
70. León, M.G.F.-D.; Duarte-Escalante, E.; Calderón-Ezquerro, M.D.C.; Jiménez-Martínez, M.D.C.; Acosta-Altamirano, G.; Moreno-Eutimio, M.A.; Zúñiga, G.; García-González, R.; Ramírez-Pérez, M.; Reyes-Montes, M.D.R. Diversity and characterization of airborne bacteria at two health institutions. *Aerobiologia* **2015**, *32*, 187–198. [CrossRef]
71. Lenart-Boron, A.; Wolny-Koładka, K.; Stec, J.; Kasprowic, A. Phenotypic and Molecular Antibiotic Resistance Determination of Airborne Coagulase Negative *Staphylococcus* spp. Strains from Healthcare Facilities in Southern Poland. *Microb. Drug Resist.* **2016**, *22*, 515–522. [CrossRef] [PubMed]
72. Mirhoseini, S.H.; Nikaeen, M.; Satoh, K.; Makimura, K. Assessment of Airborne Particles in Indoor Environments: Applicability of Particle Counting for Prediction of Bioaerosol Concentrations. *Aerosol Air Qual. Res.* **2016**, *16*, 1903–1910. [CrossRef]
73. D'Arcy, N.; Canales, M.; Spratt, D.A.; Lai, K.M. Healthy schools: Standardisation of culturing methods for seeking airborne pathogens in bioaerosols emitted from human sources. *Aerobiologia* **2012**, *28*, 413–422. [CrossRef]

Publisher's Note: MDPI stays neutral with regard to jurisdictional claims in published maps and institutional affiliations.

atmosphere

MDPI

Article

Microbiological Air Quality in a Highschool Gym Located in an Urban Area of Southern Poland—Preliminary Research

Ewa Brągoszewska [1,*], Izabela Biedroń [2] and Anna Mainka [3]

1 Faculty of Energy and Environmental Engineering, Department of Technologies and Installations for Waste Management, Silesian University of Technology, 18 Konarskiego St., 44-100 Gliwice, Poland

2 Faculty of Science, Universität Bern, Hochschulstrasse 6, 3012 Bern, Switzerland; izabiedron@gmail.com

3 Faculty of Energy and Environmental Engineering, Department of Air Protection, Silesian University of Technology, 22B Konarskiego Str., 44-100 Gliwice, Poland; Anna.Mainka@polsl.pl

* Correspondence: Ewa.Bragoszewska@polsl.pl; Tel.: +48-322-372-762

Received: 27 June 2020; Accepted: 27 July 2020; Published: 29 July 2020

check for updates

Abstract: The benefits of regular exercise include improved physical and mental health. The school gym is a particular micro-environment where students perform intensive physical training. The question is if there is an increased risk of microbiological contamination. This preliminary work studied the exposure of students to bacterial aerosol (BA) in a highschool gym located in an urban area of Southern Poland. A sampling of BA was undertaken with an Andersen six-stage impactor (ANDI). BA was identified using API (analytical profile index) tests. The BA concentrations were expressed as Colony Forming Units (CFU) per cubic metre of air. The results showed that before gym classes (BGC), the concentration of BA was $4.20 \times 10^2 \pm 49.19$ CFU/m^3, while during gym classes (DGC), the level of BA more than doubled ($8.75 \times 10^2 \pm 121.39$ CFU/m^3). There was also an increase in the respirable fraction of BA (particles less than 3.3 μm). Before the start of the sports activities, respirable fraction accounted for 30% of the BA, while during physical education classes, this share increased to over 80%. Identification of BA species showed that the dominant group of bacteria in the indoor air of the gym BGC was Gram-positive rods (61%) and for DGC it was Gram-positive cocci (81%). We detected that one bacteria strain (*Corynebacterium striatum*) was classified into risk group 2 (RG2) according to Directive 2000/54/EC. Additionally, multi-antibiotic resistance (MAR) showed that among the isolated airborne bacteria, the highest antibiotic resistance was demonstrated by *Staphylococcus epidermis* (isolated DGC) and *Pseudomonas* sp. (isolated BGC). The quantitative and qualitative information on microbiological air quality (MIAQ) in the school gym indicates that the actions to improve indoor physical activity spaces are recommended.

Keywords: microbiological indoor air quality (MIAQ); bacterial aerosol (BA); size distribution; gymnastic hall; multi-antibiotic resistance (MAR)

1. Introduction

According to available studies on indoor air quality (IAQ), it was found that both air pollution and physical conditions (including temperature, humidity and inefficient ventilation) have a negative impact on the health of building residents [1–9].

Previous studies conducted in educational buildings showed that poor microbiological indoor air quality (MIAQ) in classrooms exerts a negative effect on students' learning performance [10]. Poor air quality has been shown to increase absenteeism and increase the risk of asthma and other health-related issues [11,12]. In general, about 1% of school-age children in Poland suffer from chronic respiratory diseases [13]. There are 8000 secondary schools in Poland, with 13,360 students. The most popular schools are post-gymnasium highschools, which enable students to obtain a certificate of maturity and continue to education in universities. These schools are attended by 86.8% of all post-gymnasium students. Among the educational facilities, 3818 include highschools, 424 of which are located in the cities of an urban area of Southern Poland (Silesia Province) [14].

Regulation from the Minister of National Education and Sport on safety and hygiene in public and non-public schools and institutions, and Framework Directive 89/391/EEC [15], oblige school principals to ensure safe and hygienic conditions for students and teachers [16,17]. This requirement is supported by the framework of school statutes as well as other general health and safety regulations.

Compared to other indoor spaces in educational buildings, it is interesting to note that school gyms offer a unique place to explore microbial diversity. Sports facilities exhibit exceptional conditions for bacterial aerosol (BA) proliferation, and the conditions in which students exercise are seldom examined. One of the parameters prevalent in this type of building is moisture emitted due to perspiration and water condensation as a result of the physical activity of occupants [18]. Although regular exercise improves overall well-being, decreases the prevalence of diseases and improves physical health, the public's passion for exercise has been discouraged by severe air pollution [19]. Increased physical activity in polluted areas consequently leads to elevated exposure of some pollutants producing adverse health effects [20–22]. During exercise, the air is generally inhaled through the mouth and at a higher-than-normal rate, so the intake of airborne contaminants increases, with increased penetration to the lower parts of the lungs [12].

Regardless of the existence of many reports on MIAQ in educational buildings [2,3,11,23–26], studies on potential risks of exposure to BA in gyms situated in academic environments during physical education or exercise lessons are very limited [18,27–29]. Additionally, there is still a shortage of information on the transmission of antimicrobial resistance through the air [30]. Multi-antibiotic resistance (MAR) is considered to be a rapidly progressing global public health issue with the potential of extensive environmental transmission. It is a widespread and alarming issue in global health, causing more than 700,000 deaths every year [31]. Including information about MIAQ in indoor spaces is recommended for health and well-being [32].

The objectives of this study are: (a) to assess bacterial aerosol (BA) air quality in the gymnastic hall of a highschool building located in the urban area of Southern Poland, (b) to determine the concentration and BA particle size distribution in the gymnastic hall before gym classes (BGC), during gym classes (DGC) and in the outdoor air (OUT), (c) to identify isolated strains of bacteria BGC and DGC and (d) to determine the antibiotic resistance of isolated strains of BA.

2. Experiments

2.1. Sampling Sites

The study was carried out in a highschool gym located in an urban area of Southern Poland (50°15′44.121″ N 19°0′57.16″ E). The research was conducted during the spring season. The spring season was selected for this study because recent research of MIAQ conducted in Southern Poland indicates that the highest BA concentration is consistently found in the spring [9,11,33]. Every measurement was conducted between 7:00 and 9:00 a.m. (BGC), and 10:00–12:00 a.m. (DGC, attended by 15–17 students).

In the analyzed school gym, MIAQ is primarily ensured by means of stack ventilation and airing through open and unsealed windows. The gym is aired before classes and during breaks when students leave the hall. Following Polish legislation, the ventilation system in each educational building is checked each year and should ensure three to five air changes per hour [12]. In the gymnastic hall, deep wet cleaning was carried out once a day after the occupancy period. Table 1 presents a description of the educational building. The device used for air temperature and humidity measurement was an portable Weather Station WMR 200 (Oregon Scientific, Portland, OR, USA).

Table 1. Environmental parameters and description of the analyzed gymnastic hall.

School Localization	In the City Center, Near a Busy Street
Building, built in	1900's
Ventilation system	natural
Volume, m^3	320
Number of children	15–17
Age of students	16–18
Floor covered with	PVC (polyvinyl chloride)
Indoor temperature (°C)	19.1 ± 4.6
Outdoor temperature (°C)	16.2 ± 3.1
Indoor relative humidity (%)	28.1 ± 5.4
Outdoor relative humidity (%)	36.2 ± 7.1

2.2. Sampling and Analytical Methods

BA was collected using an Andersen six-stage impactor ANDI (Thermo Fisher Scientific, Waltham, MA, USA) with cut-off diameters of 7.0, 4.7, 3.3, 2.1, 1.1 and 0.65 µm, with constant flow rate (28.3 L/min). The sampling time was 10 min, following Nevalainen et al. [34]. The device was disinfected using 70% ethanol-immersed cotton balls between each sampling. Samples were collected on nutrient media. Tryptic soy agar (TSA, BioMaxima) was used for BA, with cycloheximide (500 mg/L, 95%, ACROS Organics™, USA) added to inhibit fungal growth.

All Petri dishes were incubated for 48 h at 36 ± 1 °C. The samples of BA were collected in the center of the gymnastic hall and taken at the height of the student's breathing zone, about 1.5 m from the ground. In total, we quantitatively analyzed 324 Petri dishes (18 measurement series for OUT, BGC and DGC) and qualitatively, we analyzed 216 Petri dishes (18 measurement series both for BGC and DGC) with biological material.

The testing of blank plates was performed per batch of prepared medium at the temperature used during the performed procedure. The blanks were not contaminated. The sampling equipment (ANDI) and laboratory equipment (laminar flow cabinet, autoclave, incubators and microscope) were regularly checked and had current certificates.

2.3. Bacteria Identification

BA strains obtained from each intake were isolated. In the first stage, colony morphology was macroscopically determined (shape, pigmentation, edges, etc.). The next stage was microscopic analysis (bacterial morphology, motility and reaction to Gram staining, etc.). The next steps focused on selecting a group of microorganisms present in each of the tested samples. For this purpose, a comparative analysis of the created feature matrix was used. A series of screening analyses led to the acquisition of strains of bacteria, present during each collection. The selected microorganisms were then identified, and their antibiotic resistance was determined.

Next, we gathered information about the main groups of bacteria present in the indoor air in the gymnastic hall. Isolated strains were cultivated on the agar medium with the addition of blood (trypticase-soy agar with 5% sheep blood). Selected strains were characterized in terms of their metabolic characteristics by using the biochemical test API (analytical profile index), which is supported by APIweb (bioMérieux, Marcy-l'Etoile, France). The following API systems were used: API 20E, API 20NE, API 50CH, API CORYNE, API STAPH and API STREP.

2.4. Multi-Antibiotic Resistance Test (MAR)

For antimicrobial susceptibility testing, the disc diffusion method was carried out according to the Kirby–Bauer Disk Diffusion Susceptibility Test Protocol [35]. Isolated strains of the BA were determined. During night cultures, the bacterial isolates were diluted to 1 McFarland (3×10^8 colony forming units/mL). 100 µL of bacterial inoculum was spread over the surface of a Mueller–Hinton agar plate (Oxoid, Columbia, MD, USA). Next, antimicrobial susceptibility testing discs (Oxoid, Columbia, MD, USA) were placed on inoculated Mueller–Hinton agar plates. 20 different antibiotics and their concentrations were chosen to take into consideration the common antibiotic resistance referred to in the literature on bacterial species. Three repetitions of each antibiotic were performed. Specific doses of the antibiotics are presented in Table 2.

Table 2. Antibiotics and their doses used in multi-antibiotic resistance test (MAR).

Group of Antibiotics	Antibiotic	Symbol/Dose (μg)
Penicillins	Amoxycillin	AML (25)
	Ampicillin	AMP (25)
Cephalosporines	Ceftazidime	CAZ (30)
	Cephalothin	KF (30)
	Cefuroxime	CXM (30)
Quinolones	Nalidic acid	NA (30)
Aminoglycosides	Amikacin	AK (30)
	Doxycycline	DO (30)
	Erythromycin	E (30)
	Gentamicin	CN (30)
	Kanamycin	K (30)
	Neomycin	N (30)
	Streptomycin	S (25)
	Tobramycin	TOB (10)
Tetracyclines	Tetracycline	TE (30)
Sulfonamides	Trimethoprim	W (5)
Rifampicins	Rifampicin	RD (30)
Other	Chloramphenicol	C (30)
	Nitrofurantoin	F (200)
	Novobiocin	NV (30)

Petri dishes with bacteria were incubated at 37 °C for 24 h. After incubation, the areas of inhibition growth were measured. A three-stage scale was used in order to assess the bacteria resistance to antibiotics: diameter of growth inhibition < 15 mm—bacterial resistance to an antibiotic, diameter of growth inhibition between 16 and 25 mm—intermediate bacterial resistance to an antibiotic and diameter of growth inhibition > 25 mm—bacteria sensitive to the antibiotic.

2.5. Statistical Analysis

The R Studio 1.2.5042 was used to perform all statistical analyses, and the ggplot2 package was used to generate all plots [36]. The presence of significant differences was determined using one-way analysis of variance (ANOVA). Pairwise *t*-test with Bonferroni correction for multiple comparisons was performed if significant results were obtained in the ANOVA test ($p < 0.05$).

3. Results and Discussion

3.1. Quantity of Bacterial Aerosol (BA) in a Highschool Gym: Before Gym Classes (BGC), during Gym

The BA concentration of the highschool gym before gym classes (BGC), during gym classes (DGC) and the outdoor air (OUT) was measured. The highest mean value of the concentration of BA was DGC ($8.75 \times 10^2 \pm 121.39$ CFU/m^3), whilst the mean concentration of bacteria BGC was $4.20 \times 10^2 \pm 49.19$ CFU/m^3. The OUT concentration of BA was $2.34 \times 10^2 \pm 36.33$ CFU/m^3. The maximum value of BA concentration was obtained DGC (3.78×10^2 CFU/m^3), and the minimum was obtained OUT (4.0 CFU/m^3). The BA concentration indoors was nearly four times the concentration outdoors. These results indicate that the source of the increased concentration DGC is simply due to the presence of students, because humans are the main source of bacterial emission indoors, and are confirmed with the data available in the literature [8,29,37]. BA contamination levels obtained in our study were lower than the threshold values of occupational exposure specified by the Expert Group on Biological Agents at the Polish Interdepartmental Commission for Maximum Admissible Concentrations and Intensities for Agents Harmful to Health in the Working Environment for public service buildings (5.0×10^3 CFU/m^3 for mesophilic bacteria) [38,39]. Comparing the values observed in our study with the limits suggested by the Commission of the European Communities (CEC) [40] indicates that the range of values obtained for DGC should be considered as moderate contamination (<2000 CFU/m^3), and also, for BGC and OUT, should be considered as average contamination (<500 CFU/m^3).

The ANOVA test was significant with F-value equal to 13.81. Based on these results, t-tests were used to determine for which variants there are significant differences. A significant difference was observed between BGC and DGC ($p = 0.0015$) and between DGC and OUT ($p = 0.00086$). No significant difference was found between OUT and BGC ($p = 0.4577$).

The Environmental Protection Agency (EPA) do not give any specific guidelines for bioaerosol concentration levels, so they are only as proposed by different governmental and private organizations [41]. Nevalainen, in 1989 [42], suggested an upper limit for bacterial aerosols ranging from 4500 to 10,000 CFU/m^3. However, research conducted by the WHO expert group on the assessment of the health risk of biological agents in the indoor environment suggests that the total concentration of microorganisms should not exceed 1000 CFU/m^3 [43].

Similar studies carried out in Poland 16 years ago showed that the level of BA before gym classes was 5.50×10^2 CFU/m^3. During the first lesson in the gym, the concentration of BA was 10 times higher (5.50×10^3 CFU/m^3) [44]. As it can be seen, the concentration of BA before gym classes is on the comparable level, but during gym classes, the study of Pastuszka et al. [44] reported significantly higher levels of BA. The probable reason was the higher occupancy in the gym.

Studies of MIAQ in fitness centers in Portugal reported that the average BA concentration was 5.56×10^2 CFU/m^3 and 8.24×10^2 CFU/m^3 in the studio and bodybuilding room, respectively. As it can be seen, the average level of BA during gym classes is in agreement with results from the bodybuilding room, while the BA concentration before gym classes is comparable to the levels in the gym studio [18]. The results of our measures BGC also agree with the studies of Dacarro et al. [27] and Grisoli et al. [28], who reported the levels of mesophilic bacteria in Italian gyms, which were 4.93×10^2 CFU/m^3 and 3.93×10^2 CFU/m^3, respectively.

Besides, temperature and relative humidity are closely associated with bacterial growth and have significant effects on microbial diffusion in the air [28,45–47]. The ASHRAE's standard recommends that indoor temperatures in the winter and summer are between 20 and 23.8 °C and 22.7 and 26.1 °C, respectively [48]. The EPA recommends that relative humidity levels indoors should be between 30% and 50% [49]. Controlling these parameters, especially relative humidity, may be an effective strategy to prevent asthma and allergy symptoms among students and teachers [50].

3.2. Particle Size Distribution of Bacterial Aerosol (BA) in a Highschool Gym: Before Gym Classes (BGC), during Gym Classes (DGC) and Outdoor Air (OUT)

Figure 1 presents the analysis of the average concentration of BA collected from the different stages of the Andersen six-stage impactor (ANDI) in the indoor and outdoor air of the school building areas.

The highest average concentration of BA in the OUT was observed on the stage with the aerodynamic diameter ranging > 7.0 μm (Figure 1C). For BGC, the highest concentration of BA was observed for particles with an aerodynamic diameter ranging from 3.3 to 4.7 μm (Figure 1A). Stages with the aerodynamic diameter ranging from 0.65 to 3.3 μm had the highest concentration of BA from indoor samples DGC (Figure 1B).

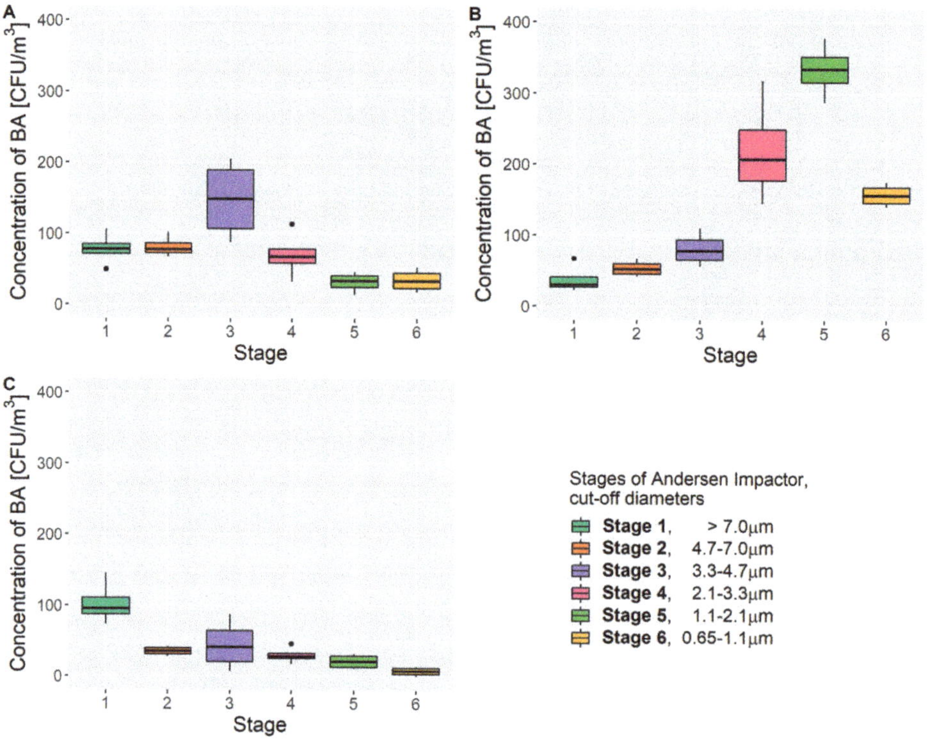

Figure 1. Average concentration of bacterial colony-forming units (CFU) per cubic meter collected from the different stages of the Andersen six-stage impactor (ANDI): (**A**) before gym classes (BGC), (**B**) during gym classes (DGC) and (**C**) in the outdoor air (OUT).

As it can be seen, the size distribution of bacteria OUT and BGC were similar. Both distributions were characterized with a large share of coarse particles of BA. However, indoor bioaerosol collected BGC indicated a little higher contribution of smaller particles and lower contribution of particles, >7.0 μm, compared to outdoor BA. The sports activity significantly changed the patterns of this size distribution, shifting the peak into the smaller BA particles—in the range from 1.1 to 3.3 μm. The size distributions of BA collected DGC might indicate that the particles of BA were relatively fresh, and generally originating from exercising students. Some studies have found that the activities of humans increase the concentrations of aerosol diameter > 1 μm [51,52] in indoor environments. We hypothesize that human activity and human presence may affect the concentration of biological particles, as they do for ordinary aerosol particles.

The results suggest that during gym classes, students are at risk of being exposed to respirable particles (less than 3.3 μm) that can reach the trachea, bronchi and alveoli, and contribute to adverse respiratory symptoms. It can be seen that the concentration levels of BA obtained in our study are below these proposed standards. However, their long-term inhalation may cause adverse health effects, especially in students sensitive to this type of air pollution.

The ratio of respirable BA during gym classes was 80% compared to the reports [53,54] of a ratio of respirable BA inside public buildings ranging between 30% and 60%. Our result is likely to be an accurate level and may be evidence for the appearance of adverse respiratory symptoms, especially in students sensitive to this type of air pollution.

On the grounds of the statistical analysis, significant differences were found between differences between BA concentration in the OUT–BGC–DGC on some stages of the Andersen six-stage impactor

(ANDI), with p-values < 0.05 (Table 3). The similar size distribution of BA we found at stage 1: between OUT and DGC, at stage 2: between OUT and BGC and BGC and DGC, at stage 3: between OUT and BGC and at stage 4, between OUT and DGC and BGC and DGC.

Table 3. Pairwise comparisons between bacterial aerosol (BA) concentrations on different stages of ANDI.

	Stage 1			Stage 2			Stage 3	
	OUT	**BGC**		**OUT**	**BGC**		**OUT**	**BGC**
BGC	0.579	-	BGC	*0.001*	-	BGC	*0.018*	-
DGC	*0.015*	0.144	DGC	0.177	*0.022*	DGC	0.718	0.134
	Stage 4			**Stage 5**			**Stage 6**	
	OUT	**BGC**		**OUT**	**BGC**		**OUT**	**BGC**
BGC	0.007	-	BGC	1	-	BGC	0.056	-
DGC	*0.001*	*0.001*	DGC	4.3×10^{-8}	6.9×10^{-8}	DGC	2.1×10^{-7}	1.2×10^{-6}

Italic entries indicate that the correlation is significant at the p-value less than 0.05; outdoor air (OUT), before gym classes (BGC) and during gym classes (DGC).

3.3. Bacterial Diversity and Antibiotic Resistance of Bacterial Aerosol (BA) in a Highschool Gym before Gym Classes (BGC) and during Gym Classes (DGC)

Detailed analysis of BA quality included 10 bacterial species (Figure 2). The statistical analysis of BA qualitative composition points to significant differences for all series between BGC and DGC for four analyzed groups of bacteria: Gram-positive cocci, non-sporing Gram-positive rods, sporing Gram-positive rods, family *Bacillaceae* and Gram-negative rods (p-values < 0.05).

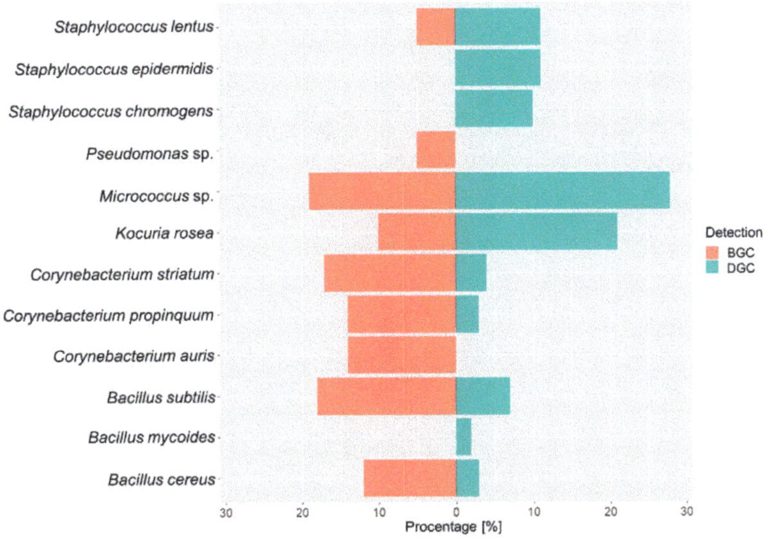

Figure 2. The most frequent BA species identified in a highschool gym before gym classes (BGC) and during gym classes (DGC).

Gram-positive cocci of the genera *Micrococcus, Kocuria* and *Staphylococcus* were the main components of the bacteria DGC. When there were no students exercising at the gym, BGC Gram-positive cocci constituted 34% of the total BA. During the sporting activity, the percentage of these bacteria increased and constituted 81%. This group of bacteria commonly occur in natural environments and colonize the surface of human skin.

DGC, three *Staphylococcus* species were identified, with a high percentage of *S. lentus*, *S. epidermidis* and *S. chromogens*. This species composition is comparable to that identified in the indoor air of preschools, primary schools and highschools during the spring in 2016 and 2017 in Poland [11]. *Staphylococcus* was also the dominant bacteria group in sports facilities at the Centre of Physical Culture and Sport at the University in Northern Poland [12]. This bacteria genus may particularly affect the health of students [55].

The most frequently isolated group bacteria BGC was Gram-positive rods. Bacteria in this group are common in samples of food, water, soil and outdoor air [45]. Many of the Gram-positive rods are found in normal skin and mucous membrane flora of humans and various animals and can cause human infections [56].

According to the classifications in Directive 2000/54/EC [57], biological agents from risk group 2 (RG2) were also detected among isolated microorganisms. It was only one strain—*Corynebacterium striatum*, for which BGC constituted 14%, while DGC constituted 4% of total microbiota. Bacteria from RG2 are associated with human disease, which is rarely serious or for which preventive and therapeutic interventions are often available.

3.4. Multi Antibiotic Resistance Test (MAR) of Bacterial Aerosol (BA) in a Highschool Gym before Gym Classes (BGC) and during Gym Classes (DGC)

Antibiotic-resistant genes are rapidly evolving into a significant environmental problem and have become a global threat to public health [58]. Results of MAR (Figure 3) can be presented as the inhibition rate of growth diameter around antimicrobial susceptibility testing disks, mean values for each antibiotic and tested strain (in millimeters). The results of MAR demonstrated that the air environment DGC was highly impacted by antibiotic resistance bacteria, while in BGC, a smaller proportion of resistant microorganisms was observed.

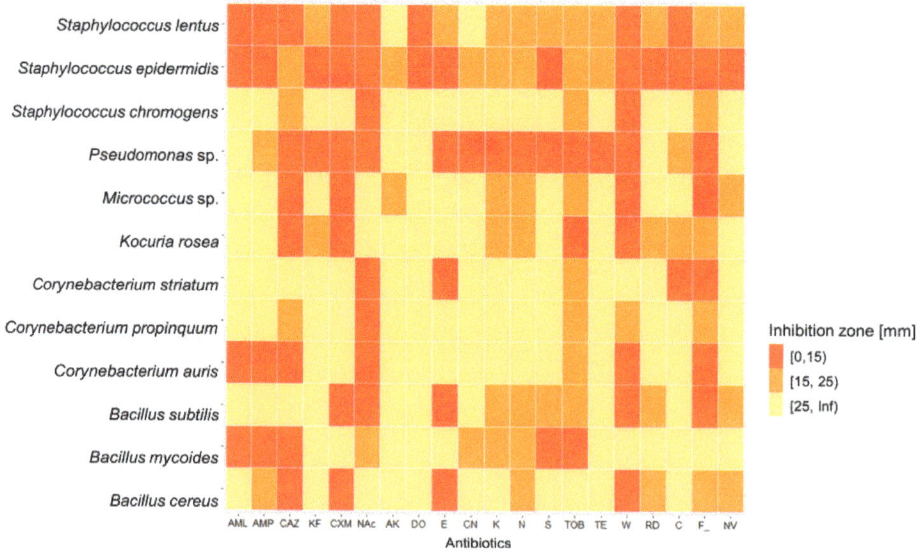

Figure 3. Results of antibiotic resistance testing. Expressed in the values of the growth inhibition zone (mm).

The highest antibiotic resistance bacteria isolated DGC was *Staphylococcus epidermis. S. epidermidis* is from a group of mannitol-fermenting coagulase-negative staphylococci characterized by multiple antibiotic resistance [59,60].

S. epidermidis was one of the isolates showing the highest antibiotic resistance. Although it is an opportunistic pathogen and the most common skin commensal [61], it plays an important role in balancing the skin microflora and serves as a source of resistance genes [62]. Despite its widespread presence, we must not forget that infections are mainly caused by endogenous microflora [63]. In the case of exercises in the gym, we can expect the appearance of abrasions or scratches among students that are the result of physical activity. It is known that this species exhibits resistance to many antibiotics, and in addition, in recent years, methicillin-resistant *Staphyloccocus epidermidis* (MRSE) is the most common of the species in medical facilities [64]. Among strains isolated in hospitals, resistance to beta-lactam antibiotics—mainly penicillin and cephalosporins—was most commonly observed [63]. The isolated strain also had such a resistance pattern.

Our attention was drawn to the fact that in hospital cases, we often talk about postoperative infections (often associated with implant placement), where high antibiotic resistance is explained by the formation of biofilms by microorganisms [62,65]. In this case, a strain with a similar resistance pattern was isolated from the air sample.

The highest antibiotic resistance bacteria isolated BGC was *Pseudomonas* sp. *Pseudomonas* species are known to harbor multiple intrinsic and acquired resistance genes and host several mobile genetic elements [66]. *Pseudomonas* sp. includes species with both clinical and environmental implications. Important members of this genus include *P. aeruginosa, P. fluorescens* and *P. stutzeri*.

However, the presence of resistant *Pseudomonas* representatives, even if they do not belong to pathogenic species, confirms the results of Kittinger, in which it has been shown that these species can be a reservoir of antibiotic resistance and in favorable conditions pass it on to pathogenic species through horizontal gene transfer [66]. It was noted that *Pseudomonas* isolates from environmental samples (freshwater) show much lower antibiotic resistance than clinical isolates [67]. In our research, the bioaerosol isolate presents a resistance pattern more similar to clinical isolates. This confirms the assumption that the source of bioaerosol emissions in the gym is mainly human.

The most sensitive bacteria to antibiotics are *Corynebacterium striatum* and *Corynebacterium propinquum* (isolated in both BGC and DGC). *Corynebacterium* species are widely distributed in the environment and in the microbiota of humans and animals [68].

The most effective antibiotics were amikacin and doxycycline (aminoglycosides group), which are on the World Health Organization list of basic medicines (the safest and most effective medicines needed in the healthcare system). Aminoglycosides are natural or semisynthetic antibiotics derived from actinomycetes. They are potent, broad-spectrum antibiotics which act by inhibiting protein synthesis [69].

4. Conclusions

Although the presented research is the result of preliminary studies, the data cover one season and a limited number of repetitions, they allow the following conclusions to be drawn:

1. Indoor level of bacterial aerosol (BA) is higher than outdoor.
2. During gym classes (DGC) concentration of BA is >500 CFU/m^3, pointing to moderate contamination.
3. The sports activity shifted the peak of this size distribution into the smaller particles (1.1 to 3.3 μm), pointing to fresh human origin particles.
4. Dominating bacterial species is Gram-positive cocci, which commonly occur on human skin.
5. Among determined biological agents, only one strain, *Corynebacterium striatum,* belongs to RG2 (risk group 2), and it constituted 14% of BA before gym classes (BCG); however, this bacteria rarely causes serious diseases.

6. DGC, the proportion of antibiotic resistance bacteria was higher than BGC.
7. The highest antibiotic resistance revealed *Staphylococcus epidermis* (isolated DGC) and *Pseudomonas* sp. (isolated BGC).
8. The most sensitive bacteria to antibiotics are *Corynebacterium striatum* and *Corynebacterium propinquum* (isolated both BGC and DGC).

The results of this study indicate that the concentrations of bacterial aerosol (BA) in a highschool gym located in the naturally ventilated historic building are not particularly hazardous for the occupants, but the air in the gym is more contaminated than outdoor air, so we recommend to perform gym classes outside the building as often as possible.

Author Contributions: Conceptualization, E.B.; Data curation, E.B. and I.B.; Methodology, E.B. and I.B.; Supervision, E.B.; Visualization, I.B.; Writing—original draft, E.B., I.B. and A.M.; Writing—review and editing, E.B., I.B. and A.M. All authors have read and agreed to the published version of the manuscript.

Funding: This work was supported by the Faculty of Energy and Environmental Engineering, Silesian University of Technology (statutory research).

Conflicts of Interest: The authors declare no conflict of interest.

References

1. Mainka, A.; Brągoszewska, E.; Kozielska, B.; Pastuszka, J.S.; Zajusz-Zubek, E. Indoor air quality in urban nursery schools in Gliwice, Poland: Analysis of the case study. *Atmos. Pollut. Res.* **2015**, *6*, 1098–1104. [CrossRef]
2. Mendell, M.J.; Heath, G.A. Do indoor pollutants and thermal conditions in schools influence student performance? A critical review of the literature. *Indoor Air* **2005**, *15*, 27–52. [CrossRef]
3. Blondeau, P.; Iordache, V.; Poupard, O.; Genin, D.; Allard, F. Relationship between outdoor and indoor air quality in eight French schools. *Indoor Air* **2005**, *15*, 2–12. [CrossRef] [PubMed]
4. Maslesa, E.; Jensen, P.A.; Birkved, M. Indicators for quantifying environmental building performance: A systematic literature review. *J. Build. Eng.* **2018**, *19*, 552–560. [CrossRef]
5. Dimitroulopoulou, C. Ventilation in European dwellings: A review. *Build. Environ.* **2012**, *47*, 109–125. [CrossRef]
6. Madsen, A.M.; Moslehi-Jenabian, S.; Islam, M.Z.; Frankel, M.; Spilak, M.; Frederiksen, M.W. Concentrations of Staphylococcus species in indoor air as associated with other bacteria, season, relative humidity, air change rate, and S. aureus-positive occupants. *Environ. Res.* **2018**, *160*, 282–291. [CrossRef]
7. Bakó-Biró, Z.; Clements-Croome, D.J.; Kochhar, N.; Awbi, H.B.; Williams, M.J. Ventilation rates in schools and pupils' performance. *Build. Environ.* **2012**, *48*, 215–223. [CrossRef]
8. Brągoszewska, E.; Palmowska, A.; Biedroń, I. Investigation of indoor air quality in the ventilated ice rink arena. *Atmos. Pollut. Res.* **2020**, *11*, 903–908. [CrossRef]
9. Brągoszewska, E.; Biedroń, I.; Kozielska, B.; Pastuszka, J.S. Microbiological indoor air quality in an office building in Gliwice, Poland: Analysis of the case study. *Air Qual. Atmos. Health* **2018**, *11*, 729–740. [CrossRef]
10. Wargocki, P.; Porras-Salazar, J.A.; Contreras-Espinoza, S.; Bahnfleth, W. The relationships between classroom air quality and children's performance in school. *Build. Environ.* **2020**, *173*, 106749. [CrossRef]
11. Brągoszewska, E.; Mainka, A.; Pastuszka, J.; Lizończyk, K.; Desta, Y. Assessment of Bacterial Aerosol in a Preschool, Primary School and High School in Poland. *Atmosphere* **2018**, *9*, 87. [CrossRef]
12. Małecka-Adamowicz, M.; Kubera, Ł.; Jankowiak, E.; Dembowska, E. Microbial diversity of bioaerosol inside sports facilities and antibiotic resistance of isolated Staphylococcus spp. *Aerobiologia* **2019**, *35*, 731–742. [CrossRef]
13. Pośniak, M.; Jankowska, E.; Kowalska, J.; Gołofit-Szymczak, M. *Kształtowanie Jakości Powietrza W Pomieszczeniach Szkolnych*; CIOP: Warszawa, Poland, 2010; ISBN 978-83-7373-095-3. (In Polish)
14. Central Statistical Office in Poland. Oświata I Wychowanie W Roku Szkolnym 2016/2017. Available online: https://stat.gov.pl/obszary-tematyczne/edukacja/edukacja/oswiata-i-wychowanie-w-roku-szkolnym-20162017,1,12.html (accessed on 13 May 2020). (In Polish)

15. EU. *Council Directive 89/391/EEC of 12 June 1989 on the Introduction of Measures to Encourage Improvements in the Safety and Health of Workers at Work.* 1989. Available online: https://eur-lex.europa.eu/legal-content/EN/ALL/?uri=CELEX%3A31989L0391 (accessed on 13 May 2020).
16. Regulation of the Minister of Higher Education Dated. Available online: http://prawo.sejm.gov.pl/isap.nsf/DocDetails.xsp?id=WDU20030060069 (accessed on 13 May 2020). (In Polish)
17. Polish Journal of Laws no. 95 Position 425 Act on the Educational System. 1991. Available online: https://www.ilo.org/dyn/natlex/natlex4.detail?p_lang=en&p_isn=92248 (accessed on 13 May 2020). (In Polish)
18. Ramos, C.A.; Viegas, C.; Verde, S.C.; Wolterbeek, H.T.; Almeida, S.M. Characterizing the fungal and bacterial microflora and concentrations in fitness centres. *Indoor Built Environ.* **2016**, *25*, 872–882. [CrossRef]
19. Ni, X.F.; Peng, S.C.; Wang, J.Z. Is morning or evening better for outdoor exercise? An evaluation based on nationwide PM2.5 data in China. *Aerosol Air Qual. Res.* **2019**, *19*, 2093–2099. [CrossRef]
20. Slezakova, K.; Peixoto, C.; Pereira, M.D.C.; Morais, S. (Ultra) Fine particle concentrations and exposure in different indoor and outdoor microenvironments during physical exercising. *J. Toxicol. Environ. Health Part A Curr. Issues* **2019**, *82*, 591–602. [CrossRef]
21. Carlisle, A.J.; Sharp, N.C. Exercise and outdoor ambient air pollution. *Br. J. Sports Med.* **2001**, *35*, 214–222. [CrossRef]
22. Qin, F.; Yang, Y.; Wang, S.T.; Dong, Y.N.; Xu, M.X.; Wang, Z.W.; Zhao, J.X. Exercise and air pollutants exposure: A systematic review and meta-analysis. *Life Sci.* **2019**, *218*, 153–164. [CrossRef]
23. Daisey, J.M.; Angell, W.J.; Apte, M.G. Indoor air quality, ventilation and health symptoms in schools: An analysis of existing information. *Indoor Air* **2003**, *13*, 53–64. [CrossRef]
24. Ross, M.A.; Curtis, L.; Scheff, P.A.; Hryhorczuk, D.O.; Ramakrishnan, V.; Wadden, R.A.; Persky, V.W. Association of asthma symptoms and severity with indoor bioaerosols. *Allergy* **2000**, *55*, 705–711. [CrossRef]
25. Andualem, Z.; Gizaw, Z.; Bogale, L.; Dagne, H. Indoor bacterial load and its correlation to physical indoor air quality parameters in public primary schools. *Multidiscip. Respir. Med.* **2019**, *14*, 2. [CrossRef]
26. Yang, W.; Sohn, J.; Kim, J.; Son, B.; Park, J. Indoor air quality investigation according to age of the school buildings in Korea. *J. Environ. Manag.* **2009**, *90*, 348–354. [CrossRef]
27. Dacarro, C.; Picco, A.M.; Grisoli, P.; Rodolfi, M. Determination of aerial microbiological contamination in scholastic sports environments. *J. Appl. Microbiol.* **2003**, *95*, 904–912. [CrossRef]
28. Grisoli, P.; Albertoni, M.; Rodolfi, M. Application of Airborne Microorganism Indexes in Offices, Gyms, and Libraries. *Appl. Sci.* **2019**, *9*, 1101. [CrossRef]
29. Canha, N.; Almeida, S.M.; Freitas, M.D.C.; Wolterbeek, H.T. Assessment of bioaerosols in urban and rural primary schools using passive and active sampling methodologies. *Arch. Environ. Prot.* **2015**, *41*, 11–22. [CrossRef]
30. Asaduzzaman, M.; Hossain, M.I.; Saha, S.R.; Islam, R.; Ahmed, N.; Islam, M.A. Quantification of airborne resistant organisms with temporal and spatial diversity in Bangladesh: Protocol for a cross-sectional study. *J. Med. Internet Res.* **2019**, *8*, e14574. [CrossRef]
31. O'Neill, J. *Tackling Drug-Resistant Infections Globally: Final Report and Recommendations;* Review on Antimicrobial Resistance; Wellcome Trust and HM Government: London, UK, 2016; pp. 1–84.
32. Andrade, A.; Dominski, F.H.; Coimbra, D.R. Scientific production on indoor air quality of environments used for physical exercise and sports practice: Bibliometric analysis. *J. Environ. Manag.* **2017**, *196*, 188–200. [CrossRef]
33. Brągoszewska, E.; Biedroń, I. Indoor Air Quality and Potential Health Risk Impacts of Exposure to Antibiotic Resistant Bacteria in an Office Rooms in Southern Poland. *Int. J. Environ. Res. Public Health* **2018**, *15*, 2604. [CrossRef]
34. Nevalainen, A.; Pastuszka, J.; Liebhaber, F.; Willeke, K. Performance of bioaerosol samplers: Collection characteristics and sampler design considerations. *Atmos. Environ. Part A Gen. Top.* **1992**, *26*, 531–540. [CrossRef]
35. Hudzicki, J. *Kirby-Bauer Disk Diffusion Susceptibility Test Protocol-2009;* ASM MicrobeLibrary, American Society for Microbiology: New York, NY, USA, 2016; pp. 1–23. Available online: https://www.asm.org/getattachment/2594ce26-bd44-47f6-8287-0657aa9185ad/Kirby-Bauer-Disk-Diffusion-Susceptibility-Test-Protocol-pdf.pdf (accessed on 12 May 2020).
36. R Studio, RS Team. *Integrated Development for R;* RStudio: Boston, MA, USA, 2015.

37. Gołofit-Szymczak, M.; Górny, R.L. Bacterial and fungal aerosols in air-Conditioned office buildings in Warsaw, Poland—The winter season. *Int. J. Occup. Saf. Ergon.* **2010**, *16*, 465–476. [CrossRef]
38. Górny, R.; Cyprowski, M.; Ławniczek-Wałczyk, A.; Gołofit-Szymczak, M.; Zapór, L. Biohazards in the indoor environment—A role for threshold limit values in exposure assessment. In *Management of Indoor Air Quality*; Dudzińska, M.R., Ed.; Taylor&Francis Group CRC Press: London, UK, 2011; pp. 1–20.
39. Górny, R.L.; Dutkiewicz, J. Bacterial and Fungal Aerosols in Indoor Environment in Central and Eastern European Countries. *Ann. Agric. Environ. Med.* **2002**, 17–23.
40. *European Collaborative Action (ECA) of the Commison of the European Communities Report No.12 Biological Particles in Indoor Environment*; Commison of the European Communities: Luxembourg, 1994.
41. Ki-Hyun, K.; Ehsanul, K.; Jahan, S.A. Airborne bioaerosols and their impact on human health. *J. Environ. Sci.* **2018**, *67*, 23–35.
42. Nevalainen, A. Bacterial Aerosols in Indoor Air. Ph.D. Thesis, University of Kuopio, Kuopio, Finland, 1989.
43. WHO. *Guidelines for Indoor Air Quality: Dampness and Mould*; WHO Regional Office for Europe: Copenhagen, Denmark, 2009; ISBN 7989289041683.
44. Pastuszka, J.S.; Wlazło, A.; Łudzeń-Izbińska, B.; Pastuszka, K. Bacterial and fungal aerosol in the school sport hall. *Ochrona Powietrza I Problemy Odpadów* **2004**, *38*, 62–66. (In Polish)
45. Flannigan, B.; Samson, R.A.; Miller, J.D. *Microorganisms in Home and Indoor Work Environments: Diversity, Health Impacts, Investigation and Control*, 2nd ed.; CRC Press: Boca Raton, FL, USA, 2011.
46. Brągoszewska, E.; Pastuszka, J.S. Influence of meteorological factors on the level and characteristics of culturable bacteria in the air in Gliwice, Upper Silesia (Poland). *Aerobiologia* **2018**, *34*, 241–255. [CrossRef]
47. McEldowney, S.; Fletcher, M. The effect of temperature and relative humidity on the survival of bacteria attached to dry solid surfaces. *Lett. Appl. Microbiol.* **1988**, *7*, 83–86. [CrossRef]
48. American Society of Heating, Refrigerating and Air Conditioning Engineers (Atlanta, Georgia). *ANSI/ASHRAE Standar 55-1992: Thermal Environmental Conditions for Human Occupancy*; ASHRAE: New York, NY, USA, 1992.
49. *US EPA Indoor Air Quality Tools For Schools*; Environmental Protection Agency: Washington, DC, USA, 2012.
50. Angelon-Gaetz, K.A.; Richardson, D.B.; Marshall, S.W.; Hernandez, M.L. Exploration of the effects of classroom humidity levels on teachers' respiratory symptoms. *Int. Arch. Occup. Environ. Health* **2016**, *89*, 729–737. [CrossRef]
51. Batterman, S.A. Characterization of particulate emissions from occupant activities in offices. *Indoor Air* **2001**, *11*, 35–48.
52. Raunemaa, T.; Kulmala, M.; Saari, H.; Olin, M.; Kulmala, M.H. Indoor air aerosol model: Transport indoors and deposition of fine and coarse particles. *Aerosol Sci. Technol.* **1989**, *11*, 11–25. [CrossRef]
53. Pastuszka, J.S.; Paw, U.K.T.; Lis, D.O.; Wlazło, A.; Ulfig, K. Bacterial and fungal aerosol in indoor environment in Upper Silesia, Poland. *Atmos. Environ.* **2000**, *34*, 3833–3842. [CrossRef]
54. Kim, K.Y.; Kim, C.N. Airborne microbiological characteristics in public buildings of Korea. *Build. Environ.* **2007**, *42*, 2188–2196. [CrossRef]
55. Kumari, H.; Chakraborti, T.; Singh, M.; Chakrawarti, M.K.; Mukhopadhyay, K. Prevalence and antibiogram of coagulase negative Staphylococci in bioaerosols from different indoors of a university in India. *BMC Microbiol.* **2020**, *20*, 211. [CrossRef]
56. Wilson, C.; Brigmon, R.L.; Knox, A.; Seaman, J.; Smith, G. Effects of microbial and phosphate amendments on the bioavailability of lead (Pb) in shooting range soil. *Bull. Environ. Contam. Toxicol.* **2006**, *76*, 392–399. [CrossRef]
57. Directive 2000/54/EC of the European Parliament and of the Council of 18 September 2000 on the Protection of Workers from Risks Related to Exposure to Biological Agents at Work. *Off. J. Eur. Communities* **2000**, *L 262*, 21–45.
58. Aslam, B.; Wang, W.; Arshad, M.I.; Khurshid, M.; Muzammil, S.; Rasool, M.H.; Nisar, M.A.; Alvi, R.F.; Aslam, M.A.; Qamar, M.U.; et al. Antibiotic resistance: A rundown of a global crisis. *Infect. Drug Resist.* **2018**, *10*, 1645–1658. [CrossRef]
59. Schaefler, S. Staphylococcus epidermidis BV: Antibiotic resistance patterns, physiological characteristics, and bacteriophage susceptibility. *Appl. Microbiol.* **1971**, *22*, 693–699. [CrossRef] [PubMed]

60. Bowden, M.G.; Chen, W.; Singvall, J.; Xu, Y.; Peacock, S.J.; Valtulina, V.; Speziale, P.; Höök, M. Identification and preliminary characterization of cell-wall-anchored proteins of Staphylococcus epidermidis. *Microbiology* **2005**, *151*, 1453–1464. [CrossRef] [PubMed]
61. Grice, E.A.; Segre, J.A. The skin microbiome. *Nat. Rev. Microbiol.* **2011**, *9*, 244–253. [CrossRef]
62. Otto, M. Staphylococcus epidermidis—The 'accidental' pathogen. *Nat. Rev. Microbiol.* **2009**, *7*, 555–567. [CrossRef]
63. Uçkay, I.; Pittet, D.; Vaudaux, P.; Sax, H.; Lew, D.; Waldvogel, F. Foreign body infections due to Staphylococcus epidermidis. *Ann. Med.* **2009**, *41*, 109–119. [CrossRef]
64. Mohanty, S.S.; Kay, P.R. Infection in total joint replacements.Why we screen MRSA when MRSE is the problem? *J. Bone Jt. Surg.* **2004**, *86*, 2668.
65. Arciola, C.R.; Campoccia, D.; Gamberini, S.; Donati, M.E.; Pirini, V.; Visai, L.; Speziale, P.; Montanaro, L. Antibiotic resistance in exopolysaccharide-forming *Staphylococcus epidermidis* clinical isolates from orthopaedic implant infections. *Biomaterials* **2005**, *26*, 6530–6535. [CrossRef]
66. Kittinger, C.; Lipp, M.; Baumert, R.; Folli, B.; Koraimann, G.; Toplitsch, D.; Liebmann, A.; Grisold, A.J.; Farnleitner, A.H.; Kirschner, A.; et al. Antibiotic resistance patterns of Pseudomonas spp. isolated from the river Danube. *Front. Microbiol.* **2016**, *7*, 586. [CrossRef] [PubMed]
67. Liew, S.M.; Rajasekaram, G.; Puthucheary, S.A.; Chua, K.H. Antimicrobial susceptibility and virulence genes of clinical and environmental isolates of Pseudomonas aeruginosa. *PeerJ* **2019**, *7*, e6217. [CrossRef] [PubMed]
68. Alibi, S.; Ferjani, A.; Boukadida, J.; Cano, M.E.; Fernández-Martínez, M.; Martínez-Martínez, L.; Navas, J. Occurrence of Corynebacterium striatum as an emerging antibiotic-resistant nosocomial pathogen in a Tunisian hospital. *Sci. Rep.* **2017**, *7*, 9704. [CrossRef] [PubMed]
69. Krause, K.M.; Serio, A.W.; Kane, T.R.; Connolly, L.E. Aminoglycosides: An overview. *Cold Spring Harb. Perspect. Med.* **2016**, *6*, a027029. [CrossRef] [PubMed]

atmosphere

MDPI

Article

Microclimate in Rooms Equipped with Decentralized Façade Ventilation Device

Ewa Zender-Świercz

Department of Building Physics and Renewable Energy, Faculty of Environmental Geomatic and Energy Engineering, Kielce University of Technology, 25-314 Kielce, Poland; ezender@tu.kielce.pl

Received: 29 June 2020; Accepted: 27 July 2020; Published: 29 July 2020

check for updates

Abstract: Many building are characterized by insufficient air exchange, which may result in the symptoms of sick building syndrome (SBS). A large number of existing buildings are equipped with natural ventilation, whose work is disturbed by activities going to energy-saving. The thermomodernization activities are about mounting new sealed windows and laying thermal isolation, which reduces the amount of infiltrating/exfiltrating air. In many cases, the mechanical ventilation cannot be used due to a lack of a place in building or architectural and construction requirements. One of the solutions to improve the indoor microclimate is the decentralized façade ventilation. In the article, the internal air parameters in an office room equipped with decentralized façade ventilation device were analyzed. The room was equipped with a decentralized façade unit, which cyclically supplied and removed air from the room. The time of the supply/exhaust was changed to 2 min, 4 min, and 10 min. The temperature and the humidity of the indoor air and the outdoor air and the concentration of carbon dioxide inside the room were measured. The analysis showed that despite the lack of a heater in the device, the air temperature in the workplace and in the central point of the room was in the range of 20–22 °C. The air humidity was in the range of 27–43%.

Keywords: indoor microclimate; decentralized façade ventilation; air quality

1. Introduction

In order to live a healthy life and stay in good shape, people need air with adequate parameters that is free from any pollution. Air quality also affects the learning efficiency and labor productivity of people using rooms [1–10].

The general trend today is to make buildings energy-efficient, which is understood by the majority of building administrators as a reduction in the thermal losses and heating costs. As a result of this, actions are undertaken to seal and thermally insulate the building fabric and partitions. These procedures restrict air exchange in a room equipped with natural ventilation [11,12]. A reduced volume of air entering a building negatively affects the indoor air quality and induces a rise in the temperature, humidity, and pollution volume. This situation may result in the occurrence of mold on division walls, which in turn is destructive for the structure, and fungi spores may induce allergies and asthma. According to the analysis carried out by R. Górny [13], they are in fact biologically harmful due to immune reactivity, cytotoxicity, or the transport of mycotoxins.

Poor indoor air quality results in the occurrence of sick building syndrome (SBS) symptoms. Fisk et al. [14] analyzed the impact of the ventilation system capacity on the occurrence of the SBS symptoms. The average frequency of symptom occurrence increased by 23% with a ventilation system capacity drop from 36 to 18 m^3/h·person, and it decreased by ca. 29% for air flow increase from 36 to 90 m^3/h·person. Moreover, the researchers in [15–17] have proven the dependence between the occurrence of SBS and gender. In the same thermal environments and with the same type of performed work, women complained about their health problems more often. Females are more sensitive than males to a deviation from an optimal temperature (thermal dissatisfaction ratio equals 1.74 [18,19]). For example, the adjusted odds ratio of a headache for females is 3.64 more often than for males [20].

Poor indoor air quality affects the disease incidence rate as well as work and learning efficiency [21]. The analysis conducted by Lan et al. [22] of the number of mistakes made during attention tests showed that the morning test had less mistakes than the last lesson test. Roelofsen [23] showed a productivity increase of 10 per cent when the indoor environment improved. Many researchers are interested in the analysis of dependencies between the capacities of ventilation systems and learning efficiency, for example, D. L. Johnson et al. [24], whose studies proved air quality disturbances in elementary schools and observed a carbon dioxide concentration equal to 4751 ppm. Vimalanathan and Babu [25] showed that temperature was the main factor affecting work efficiency and 21 °C was optimal, and the optimal illumination was 1000 lux.

Considering the current trend to isolate the building envelope, it is necessary to control the air humidity. The amount of moisture produced in a room (by breathing and evaporation of sweat) may even reach 100 kg per week [26]. The water vapor cannot diffuse in a sealed envelope and the air humidity increases. At the same time, the share of moisture volume in air (moisture penetrating through partitions by diffusion) in the humidity balance, determined according to the standard PN-EN 13788 [27], ranges from 1% to 3% of total moisture emission [28]. An intense removal of moisture from inside is required to maintain air humidity in a room at more or less constant level [29].

Analyses completed so far [12] have proven a growth in indoor air humidity after being thermally modernized in a naturally ventilated building. This means that while trying to reduce heat loss, the investors undertake actions affecting indoor air parameters such as humidity or pollution concentration. When any changes are to be introduced in a building, there is an unambiguous need to look globally at the building as a whole: the structure with building services. Without any extra ventilation holes provided, the indoor air humidity in rooms naturally ventilated with thermally insulated partitions increases as the moisture is not exhausted with the air to the outside, which proves an insufficient air exchange. The analysis showed that this parameter becomes higher in rooms where people are the only source of moisture, thus it can be concluded that higher humidity is not the effect of a specific office space use. It is also connected with mold species not appearing in kitchens, bathrooms, or social rooms. In buildings where thermal insulation was provided and the air supply method was altered, the air humidity remained at the same level.

Insufficient air exchange ratio in rooms increases both the humidity of the air and the carbon dioxide concentration [30]. However, greater exchange of air in naturally ventilated facilities is not an ideal solution, since it may result in an inside temperature drop [10].

Mechanical ventilation systems are most effective from the point of view of the volume of air exchanged in buildings. However, their use entails greater construction and operating costs. Heat recovery or mixing fresh air streams with exhaust air at a specific recirculation rate can be used to reduce costs, however, in each case, natural ventilation will be a cheaper solution. Researchers [31] have carried out an analysis of the natural ventilation in office buildings introduced as a solution to reduce energy consumption. The conclusion of their analysis was that sufficient air exchange in facilities equaled 1–6 h^{-1}. However, there were certain conditions here: in the building, there were great heat gains and the building was designed in consideration of the relationship between architecture, shape of the building, its location, and the effectiveness of natural ventilation. Only these buildings will not be subjected to excessive chilling.

In the case of using mechanical exhaust ventilation, the risk of inside temperature drop is even greater due to larger volumes of inflowing air. Supply and supply–exhaust ventilation systems are the only ones that allow for the control of inflow air temperature. However, in these solutions, flowing air can be perceived as an unpleasant sensation of draught (DR: draught rating) [32]; whereas the discontent of people staying in rooms increases with growing air velocity and intensity of turbulence [33]. Analyses by Toftum et al. [34] indicated that air flow from the bottom and the front at an inside temperature of 20 °C caused greater discomfort than air flow in the upper part of a room. At the same time, no discomfort was observed when the air temperature in a room was 26 °C.

Moreover, the problem of insufficient volume of air delivered to a room usually occurs in already existing facilities undergoing thermal modernization. In many cases, a mechanical ventilation system cannot be installed due to design constraints or insufficient space to fit air ducts. In this case, decentralized façade ventilation can help as it may contain units designed to alternately provide air supply and exhaust.

The literature provides analyses of decentralized façade ventilation units [35–37]; however, they usually concern the energy efficiency of a unit and its impact on building energy balance. However, it is necessary to carry out an analysis of the dependence between the inside and outside temperature in facilities equipped with decentralized façade ventilation systems.

Gruner M. and Haase M. [38] evaluated decentralized façade ventilation units with regard to their capacity to maintain thermal comfort. Temperature values measured by the authors ranged from 22 to 26 °C. However, the units analyzed by them were equipped with water heaters and heat recovery exchangers. Moreover, these units worked in pairs: one responsible for air supply and the other for exhaust.

The literature lacks analyses of solutions working not in pairs, but individually, as in some existing buildings, it is not possible to fit units working in pairs on the opposite external walls. Additionally, all of the units described in the literature have either been equipped with air heaters or a heat recovery system. Moreover, the researchers did not analyze the humidity changes in rooms equipped with decentralized façade ventilation units. The article presents an attempt to evaluate the microclimate parameters (indoor air temperature and humidity) in rooms provided with decentralized façade ventilation units.

2. Experiments

The analysis covered an office room (Figure 1) sized 2.97 m × 3.21 m × 3 m, designed for two people. The building was located in Poland in a moderate climate zone with low winter temperatures and high summer temperatures. The outdoor air temperatures characteristic for this location and at the season are within −20 to +10 °C. During the tests, the outdoor air temperature ranged from −9 to +10 °C. The heating system was deactivated in the analyzed room. Measuring equipment was located in the workplace and at the central point of the room. The room was equipped with a decentralized façade unit that was cyclically supplying and removing air from the room. During the supply cycle, air was drawn from the outside and delivered by the unit to the room, and then removed through a gap in the bottom part of the internal door. During the exhaust cycle, air was removed through the unit, and supplied via the gap in the internal door. A temperature of 21 °C was maintained in an adjacent room. The air supplied by the unit had the same temperature as the outside air, and the air flowing in through the door gap had the temperature of the air in the adjacent room.

The decentralized façade unit (Figure 2) was equipped with one fan (1) pumping air continuously in one direction, and the alternation of cycles was effected by dampers (3–6) opening and closing in pairs. Air flow route was dependent on the damper opening. Dampers 4 and 6 were open during the supply cycle, and dampers 3 and 5 were open during the exhaust cycle. During the supply cycle, the air flowed through sections 7 and 9, and during the exhaust cycle, through sections 8 and 10. Component no. 2 is an intake vent/exhaust vent, and no. 11 is the air-intake/air-exhaust.

Air temperature and humidity was measured in the room and outside. The research took 26 weeks during the fall–winter–spring seasons (from November to March). The period was divided into a two-week series, during which the measurement was performed continuously every 10 s. During the experiment, the unit setting was 2 min for eight weeks, 4 min also for eight weeks, and 10 min for 10 weeks. This research period was selected because the measurements were carried out in rooms used in real conditions (in summertime users often open windows, which considerably affects the results). Two air quality meters from Sensotron (Kozielska Street 63/5, Gliwice, Poland) were used for the tests

(Figure 3). Table 1 shows their measurement ranges and resolutions of indications. The instruments were set in the room user's workplace (on the desk) 0.8 m above the floor (point 1) and at central point of the room 1.5 m above the floor (point 2). In Figure 1, the green color indicates the location of the air supply/exhaust hole; orange indicates the locations of indoor air quality monitors; blue shows the locations of the microclimate meters; and purple represents the locations of the gap in the inner door. Figure 1 also shows the heights of the places of the measurements.

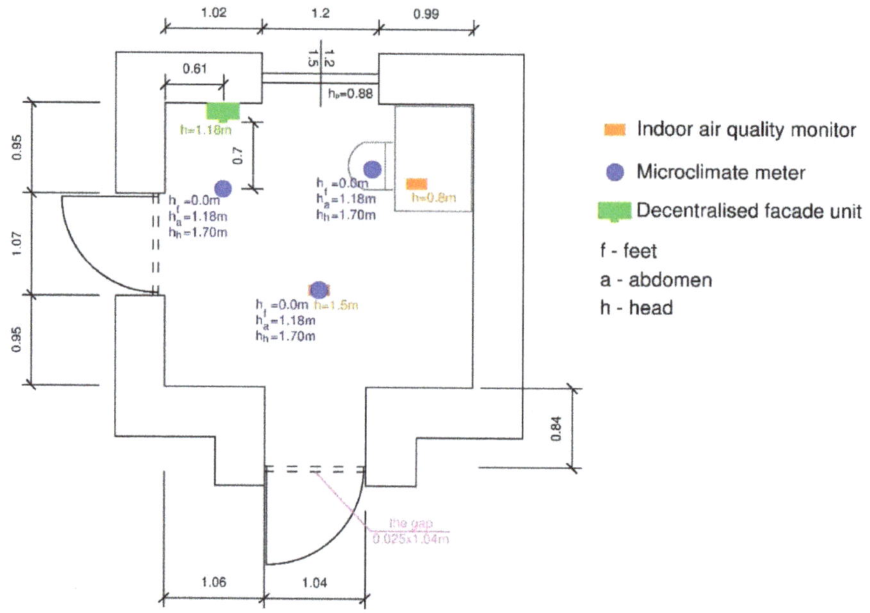

Figure 1. Layout of meters and the decentralized façade unit in the analyzed room.

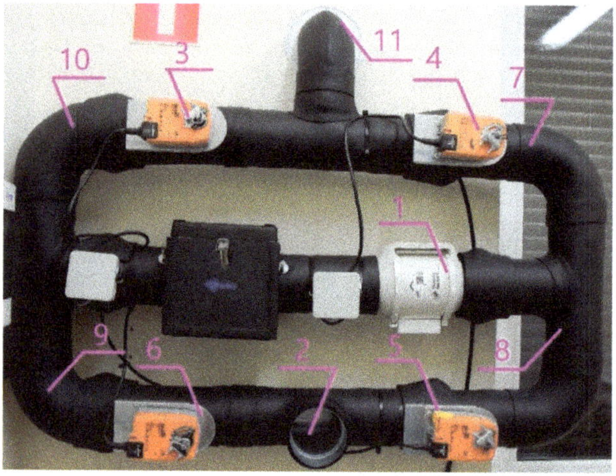

Figure 2. Wall-mounted decentralized façade ventilation unit.

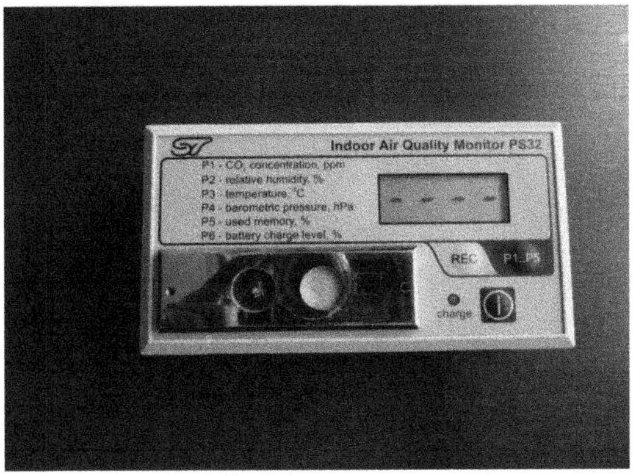

Figure 3. Indoor air quality monitor.

Table 1. Measurement ranges and resolution of indications. Indoor air quality monitor.

Parameter	Measurement Range	Resolution of Indications	Unit	Accuracy
Temperature	10–45	0.1	°C	±0.5
Humidity	0–100	0.1	%	±2
Carbon dioxide concentration	0–5000	1	ppm	±(20 + 3% of meas. value)

The air velocity in the room was measured using a microclimate meter equipped with three anemometers (Table 2). The measurement was carried out at three points: at the workplace, in the central point of the room, and 70 cm from the supply/exhaust grate. The air velocity was measured at three levels: feet, abdomen, and head.

Table 2. Microclimate meter specifications.

Parameter	Measurement Range	Resolution of Indications	Unit	Accuracy
Air velocity	0–5	0.01	m/s	±0.05 + 0.05 × Va for 0–1 m/s ±5% for 1–5 m/s
Radiant temperature	−20–50	0.01	°C	±0.4 °C

The values of the outside parameters (temperature and humidity of the external air) were recorded by a weather station located on the roof of the building. Table 3 presents the weather station specifications.

Table 3. Weather station specifications.

Parameter	Measurement Range	Resolution of Indications	Unit	Accuracy
Temperature	−40–65	0.1	°C	0.5
Humidity	1–100	1	%	3% RH; 4% over 90%

The amount of the supply/exhaust air and the supply/exhaust air velocity was measured using a balometer (Table 4).

The room ventilation unit was worked in three cycles with different air supply/exhaust duration: 2 min, 4 min, and 10 min. The time can be set in the range of 1 min to 10 min, thanks to the use of an actuator in the installation that closed and opened the dampers. The selected cycle lengths were dictated by the desire to show the differences in creating the microclimate at different settings of the device. One cycle consisted of successive air supply and exhaust. In the case of a 2 min cycle, the supply duration is 2 min. After this time, the actuator opens the closed dampers and closes the opened ones. The device switches to the exhaust air function, which also lasts 2 min. The same is applied for each time setting.

Table 4. The specifications of balometer station.

Parameter	Measurement Range	Resolution of Indications	Unit	Accuracy
Volumetric flow rate	42–4250	1	m^3/h	±3% read out value ± 12 m^3/h > 85 m^3/h
Air speed	0.125–12.5	0.01	m/s	±3% read out value ± 0.04 m/s > 0.25 m/s
Temperature	−40–121	0.1	°C	±0.3% °C
Humidity	5–95	0.1	%	±3% RH

Statistical Analysis

The unit work was evaluated from the statistical point of view. The two-factor ANOVA with replication and the Tukey multiple comparison method were employed for this purpose. Determinants for the group of comparisons included setting (air supply/exhaust duration), measuring instrument location, outside temperature, and outside humidity.

3. Results and Discussion

3.1. Experimental Studies

The air temperature measured with a 10 s step allowed for the average value for each hour for a two week period to be calculated. The average air temperature values calculated for different points of the room proved to be insignificant fluctuations at different outside air temperatures.

Figure 4 shows the average air temperature values measured at two locations in the room during thirteen two-week periods. Each line corresponds to the daily changes in the average air temperature. Each point corresponds to the mean calculated for each hour of the day from the two-week measurement period. The trajectory of changes in the analyzed parameter in time show minor daily temperature fluctuations in each of the two measurement points. During periods 1–4, the duration of the air ventilation unit supply/exhaust cycle was 2 min (2 min for air supply, and the next 2 min for air exhaust); during periods 5–8, it was 4 min; and during periods 9–13, it was 10 min.

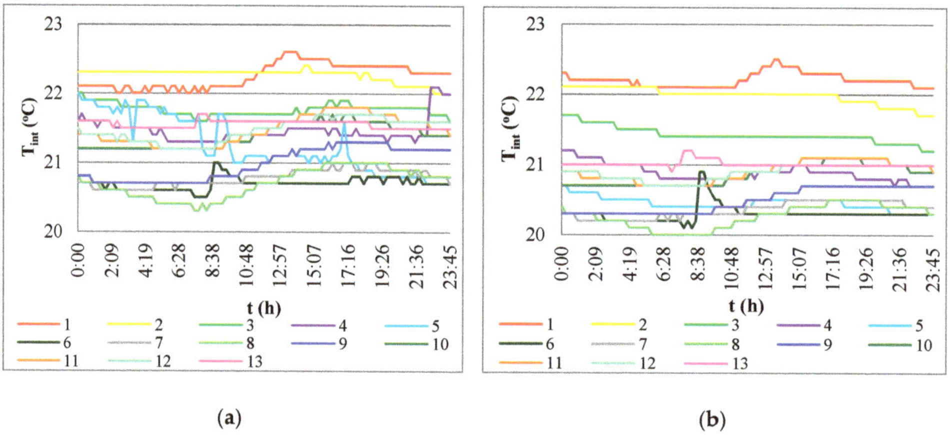

Figure 4. Average air temperature values at two locations in the room: (**a**) workplace, (**b**) central point of the room; T_{int}—inside temperature, °C; t—time, h:min.

An average of the values of measured temperature for a given hour in a day was calculated for each of the cycles, and inside air temperature values were compared to the outside air temperatures (Figure 5).

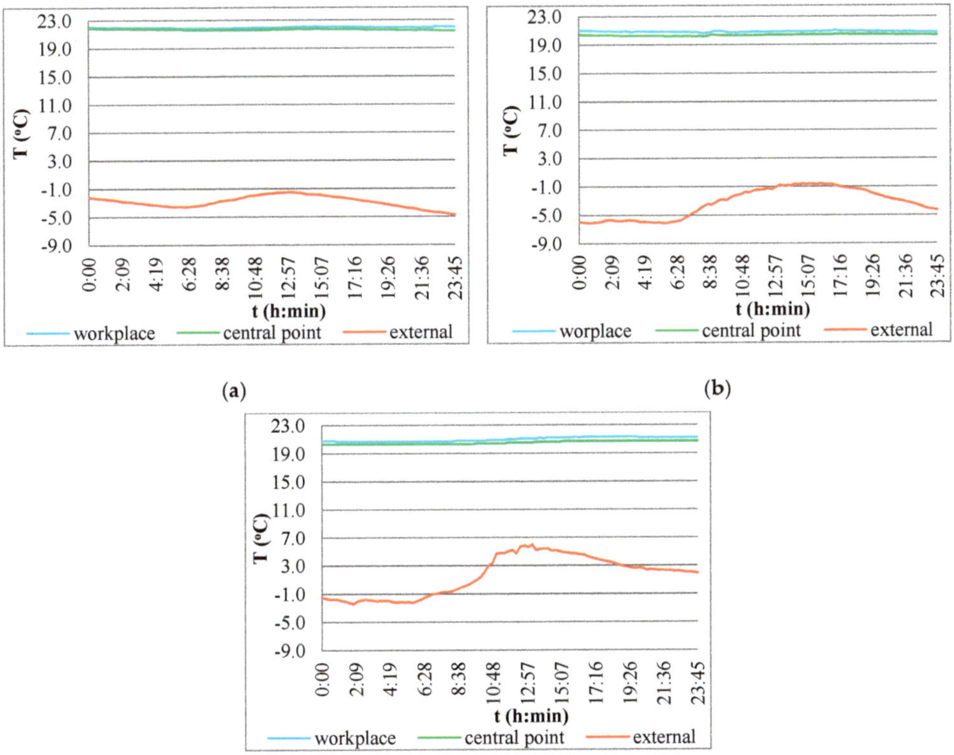

(a) (b)

(c)

Figure 5. The dependence between the average outside air temperature and average value of the parameter inside the room: (**a**) setting: 2 min, (**b**) setting: 4 min, (**c**) setting: 10 min; T—temperature, °C; t—time, h:min.

Temperature analysis proved that the values obtained for the workplace and central point of the room satisfied thermal comfort requirements according to the PN-EN 16798-1:2019-06 standard [39], despite the different values of outside air parameter. No influence of outside air temperature on room chilling was observed.

The next step involved the analysis of inside air temperature dependence on outside air temperature. Figure 6 demonstrates the obtained results and analyzed whether air supply/exhaust duration would affect the temperature value. The inside air temperature remained within the thermal comfort range throughout the measurement period. The average of the recorded temperature values ranged from 20.2 °C to 22.1 °C, which means that despite supplying low temperature air and regardless of air supply process duration (2 min, 4 min, 10 min), the temperature in the room was stable.

Both in the shortest cycle of 2 min and the longest cycle of 10 min, the values of internal air temperature met the requirements of thermal comfort (Figures 7 and 8). The thermal comfort temperatures inside the room were maintained both at the outside air temperature of 4–5 °C and the temperature of −6 °C. At the same time, the temperature of the inside air was lower in the case of the negative values of the outside temperature, but also in this case the values met the comfort requirements.

Examples of days with similar external conditions (temperature −2 ± 4 °C and humidity 80–90%) were selected from the measurement data. Figure 9 shows the course of the temperature changes over time for two locations of the meters: the workplace and the central point of the room. In both cases, the room met the requirements of thermal comfort regardless of the duration of the cycle. At the same time, the temperatures were lower for the longer cycle than for the shorter.

Average air humidity values measured at different locations in the room proved to be minor fluctuations.

Figure 10 demonstrates the fluctuations of the average air humidity values over time.

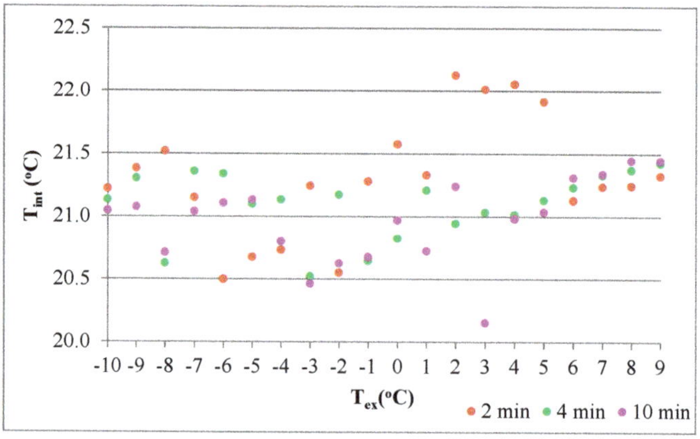

Figure 6. The dependence between inside air temperature and outside air temperature; T_{int}—inside temperature, °C; T_{out}—outside temperature, °C.

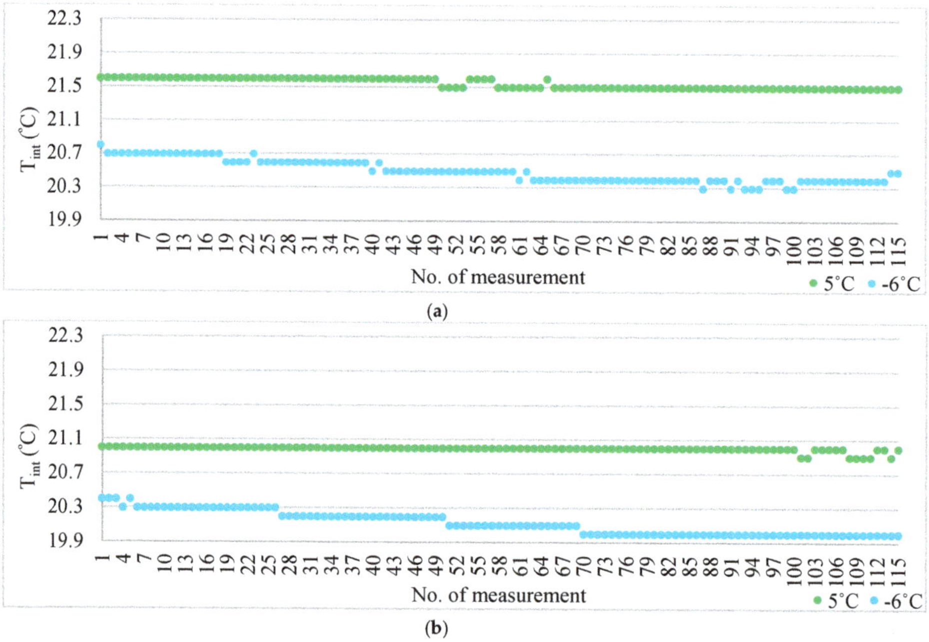

Figure 7. The course of changes in the indoor air temperature during the 10-min supply/exhaust cycle. (**a**) workplace; (**b**) central point.

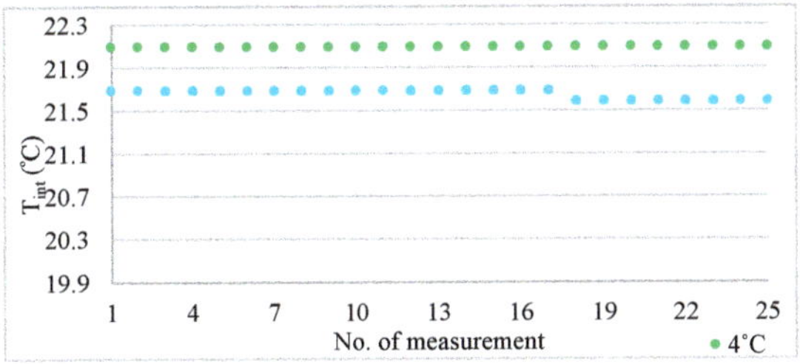

(a)

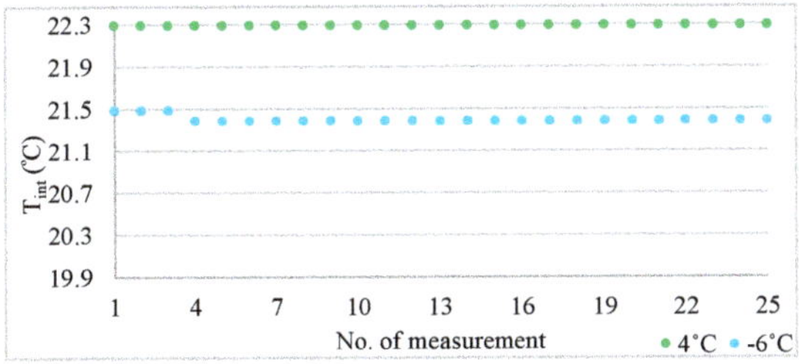

(b)

Figure 8. The course of changes in the indoor air temperature during the 2-min supply/exhaust cycle. (**a**) workplace; (**b**) central point.

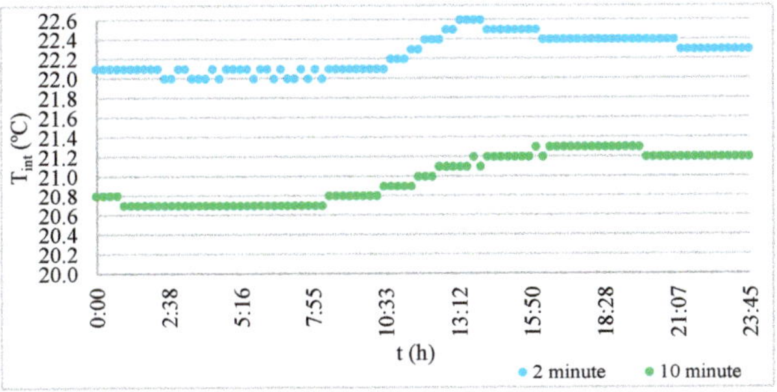

(a)

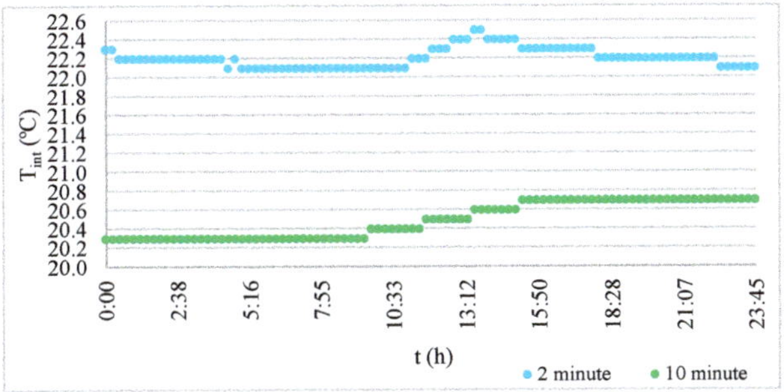

(b)

Figure 9. The course of changes in the indoor air temperature for an example day. (**a**) workplace; (**b**) central point.

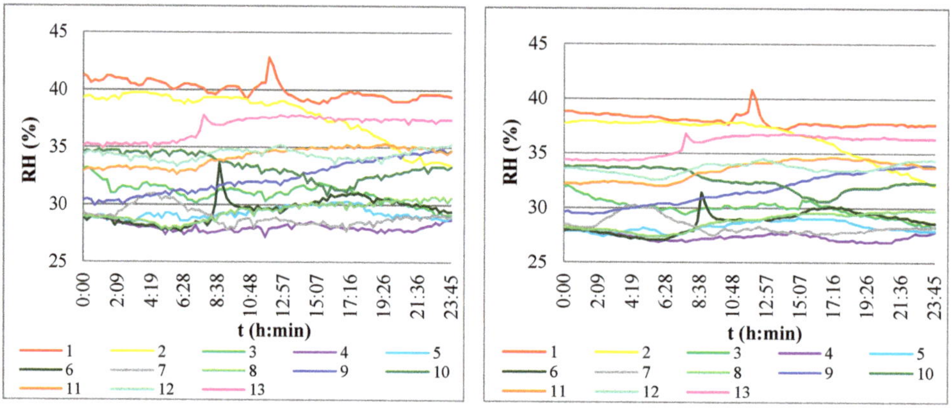

(a) **(b)**

Figure 10. Average air humidity values at two locations in the room: (**a**) workplace, (**b**) central point of the room; RH—humidity, %; t—time, h:min.

Inside air humidity values were compared to outside air humidity in each of the thirteen measurement periods (Figure 11).

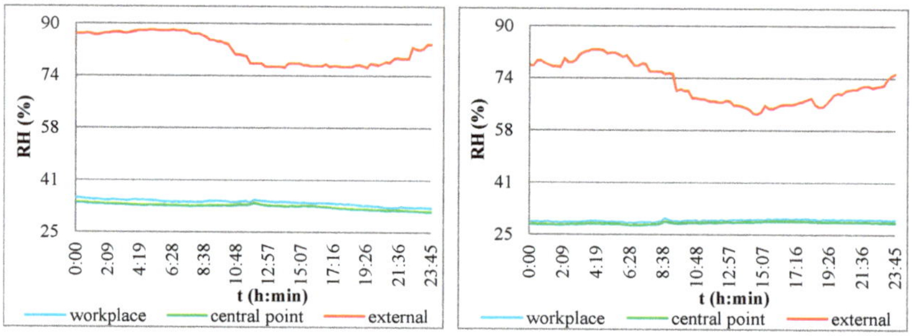

(**a**) (**b**)

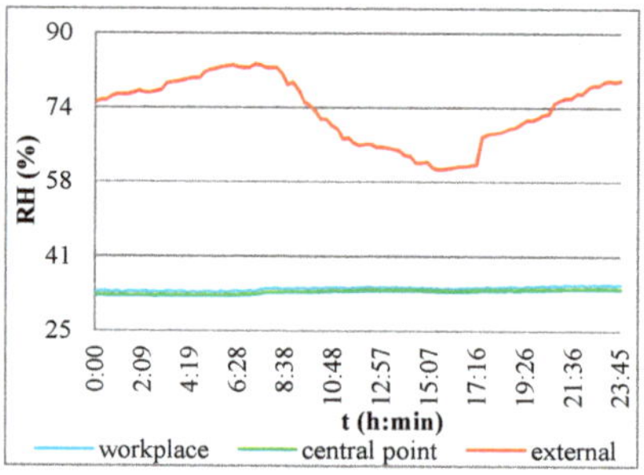

(**c**)

Figure 11. The dependence between the average outside air humidity and average value of the parameter inside the room: (**a**) setting: 2 min, (**b**) setting: 4 min, (**c**) setting: 10 min; RH—humidity, %; t—time, h:min.

Air humidity analysis proved that the values measured in the room did not always satisfy thermal comfort requirements according to the PN-EN 15251:2012 standard [40]. The decrease in the relative humidity in the room was observed when the outside temperature was low and the external relative humidity was high.

Figure 12 shows the relationship between the relative humidity of the indoor air and the temperature of the outdoor air. An increase in the indoor air humidity, along with an increase in outdoor temperature was demonstrated. Moreover, when the external temperature equaled −10 to −5 °C, the indoor air humidity did not meet the requirements of thermal comfort in accordance with PN-EN 15251:2012 [40]. At the same time, the difference between the relative humidity at the two measurement points was small.

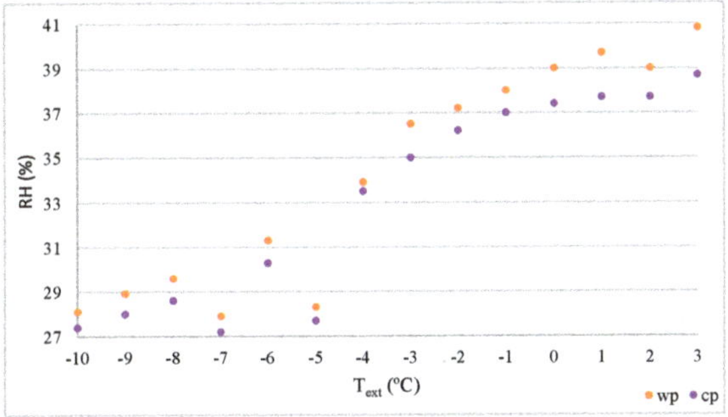

Figure 12. The relationship of the relative humidity of indoor air on the outdoor air temperature.

The device effectiveness was assessed on the basis of measurements of the supply air velocity and the level of carbon dioxide concentration. The velocity and the supply air stream were measured for each of the analyzed cycles (Figure 13). The measured values made it possible to determine the air change rate, which was 2.3 h^{-1} for the shortest cycle, and 2.7 h^{-1} for the longest cycle. For comparison, devices with heat recovery exchangers and reversible fans [41] exchange the air with an air change rate of 0.18 h^{-1}. This could be a sufficient value for living quarters, but for an office room, the number of air changes should be higher.

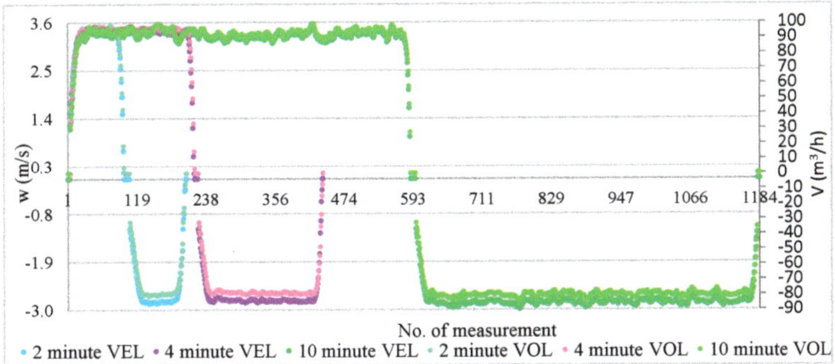

Figure 13. The course of the air velocity and air volume changes in the supply/exhaust grate during the supply and exhaust cycle.

The literature [42] shows the influence of the pressure difference inside and outside the building on the speed of the supplied air, and thus the amount of air. In the case of the presented analysis, the focus was on measuring the air velocity and amount of air flowing into the room without analyzing the impact of wind conditions on the work of the device.

The air velocity was also measured within the room at three levels: the feet, abdomen, and head. The measurement was carried out in the workplace, at a central point, and at a distance of 70 cm from the supply/exhaust grate. The performed measurements made it possible to calculate the PMV index (predicted mean vote) in accordance with the PN-EN 7730 [43] standard (Figures 14 and 15).

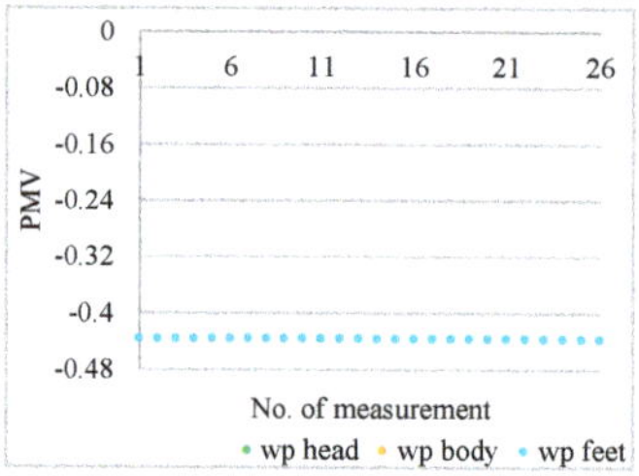

(**a**)

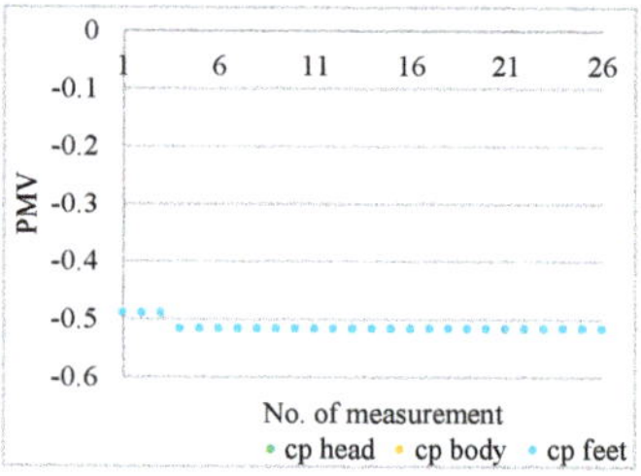

(**b**)

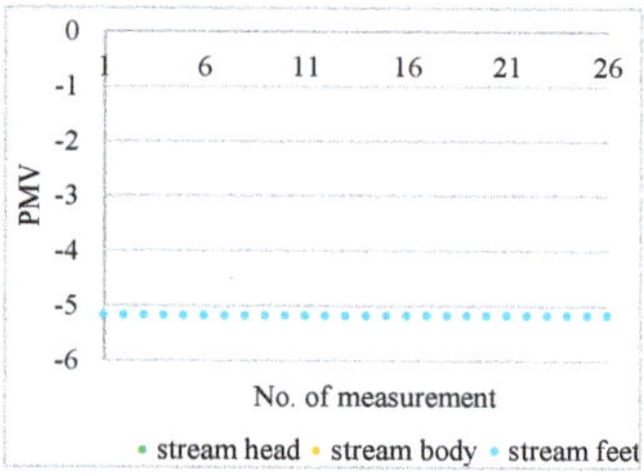

(**c**)

Figure 14. The course of changes in the predicted mean vote (PMV) indicator during the 2-min cycle airflow. (**a**) workplace, (**b**) central point of the room, (**c**) 70 cm from the air supply grate; wp: workplace; cp: central point.

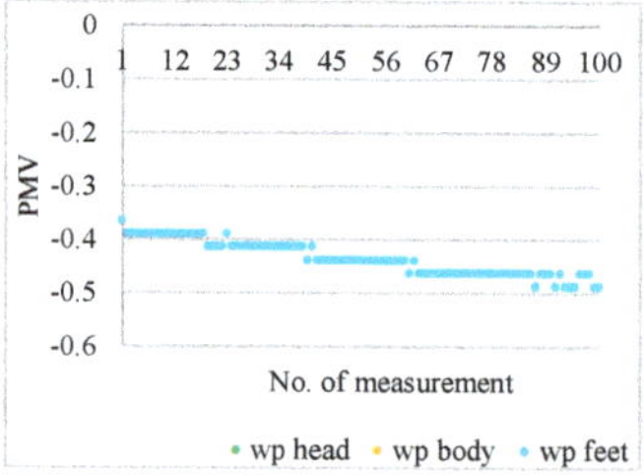

(**a**)

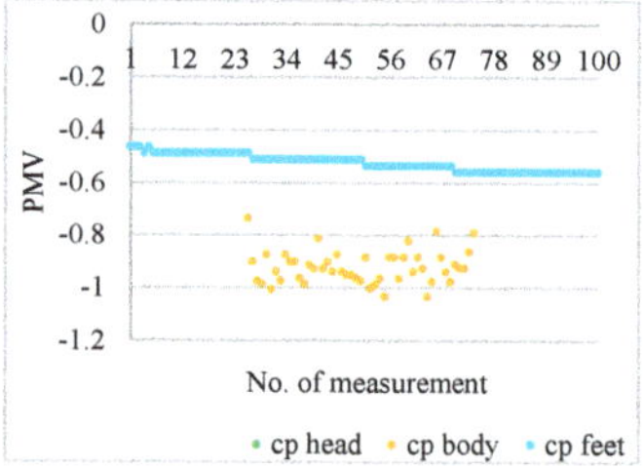

(**b**)

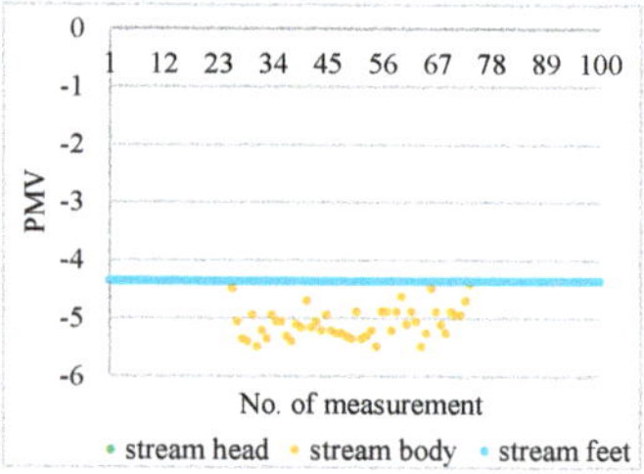

(**c**)

Figure 15. The course of changes in the PMV indicator during the 10-min cycle airflow. (**a**) Workplace, (**b**) central point of the room, (**c**) 70 cm from the air supply grate; wp: workplace; cp: central point.

On the basis of Figures 14 and 15, it can be seen that in the area of the head, abdomen, and feet, the workplace belongs to the category of room B, according to the classification of the standard PN EN 7730 [43]. The central point of the room was in category C at the end of the cycle (2 min). In the long cycle (10 min), it belonged to category C for almost the entire duration of the airflow (at all parts of the body). Additionally, the DR (draught rating) was calculated, which defines the percentage of people dissatisfied with the air movement. The analysis showed that in the case of the longest cycle (i.e., with a supplytime of 10 min), for half the time of supply (5 min), in the center of the room at the level of the abdomen, 13–20% of people were dissatisfied with the draught. However, users did not experience any draught in the area of the feet and head, so there will be no feeling of draught at every level of the body in the workplace location. However, at a distance of 70 cm from the supply/exhaust grate at the level of the abdomen, the air movement was strongly felt and the DR was from 37 to 64%. For this location, there was no feeling of draught at the levels of the feet and head. For a 2-min cycle, the index was 0 for all locations and all body parts, which means that there will be no dissatisfied people with the draft.

In the literature [44], there are efficiency analyses of decentralized devices equipped with two fans. For the efficiency assessment, we used the level of carbon dioxide concentration and radon concentration in the room. The analysis showed that the decentralized devices diluted the gaseous pollutants sufficiently. In the presented case, the measurement of carbon dioxide concentration also showed (Figure 16) that the façade device sufficiently exchanged the air for fresh air.

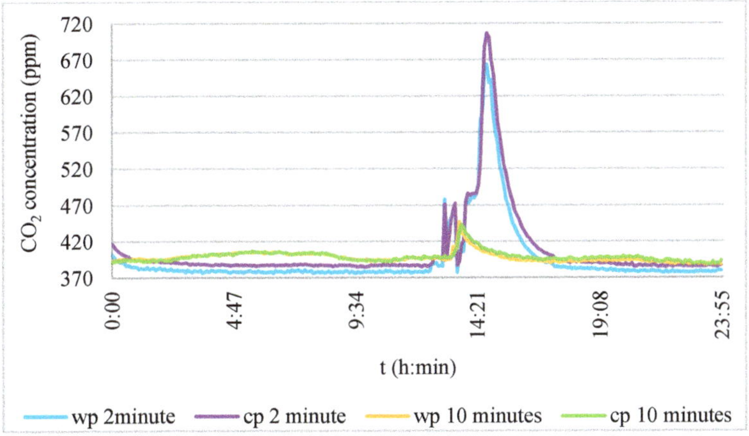

Figure 16. The course of changes in the concentration of carbon dioxide. Blue and purple colors are the 2 min cycle; yellow and green colors are the 10 min cycle; wp: workplace; cp: central.

The results are presented for an example day. There was a visible increase in the concentration of carbon dioxide upon entering the user's room. At the same time, with a longer supply/exhaust time (10 min), the maximum value of the carbon dioxide concentration was lower than for the short cycle (2 min). For each cycle length, throughout the entire period of measurements, the concentration of carbon dioxide did not exceed the value of 800 ppm, which means that the room met the ASHRAE [45] requirements for air quality in offices.

3.2. Statistical Analysis

Measured data were used to carry out the statistical analysis of the unit operation. The two-factor ANOVA was carried out for the *temperature* characteristic. The grouping variables were: *setting* with values of 2, 4, and 10 min, and *location* with values: wp (workplace) and cp (central point).

The zero hypotheses stating equality of the average values of the *temperature* characteristic was verified on the basis of all combinations of levels for both equivalent factors and the F statistic was used for this purpose (the ratio of intergroup variance to intragroup variance). Table 5 contains the results of completed calculations used to verify the hypothesis stating equality of the average values of the *temperature* characteristic in groups determined on the basis of both factors.

Table 5. Analysis of variance for the *temperature* characteristic.

Variability	Degrees of Freedom	Sum of the Squares	Mean Square	Value F	Value p
Intergroup	5	7.7	1.5	81.3	<0.0001
Intragroup	30	0.6	0.02		
Total	35	8.2			

A value p obtained for statistic F in a completed test of less than 0.0001 allows for the statement that there were at least two groups where the average values of the *temperature* characteristic differed.

Figure 17 demonstrates in box plots the significance of the effect of the interactions between the factors. The distribution of the *temperature* characteristic in groups defined by *setting* and *location* factors is illustrated in this way.

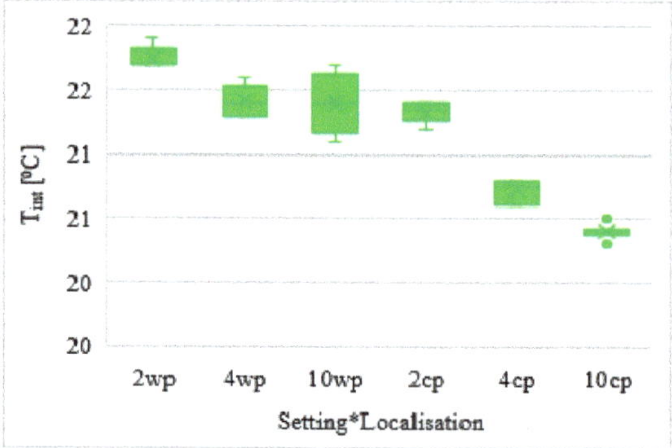

Figure 17. Box plots illustrating the distribution of the *temperature* characteristic in groups defined by pairs of factors: *setting* and *location*; T_{int}—temperature, °C; wp: workplace; cp: central point.

Figure 18 shows box plots illustrating the distribution of the *temperature* characteristic in groups defined by the *setting* factor levels.

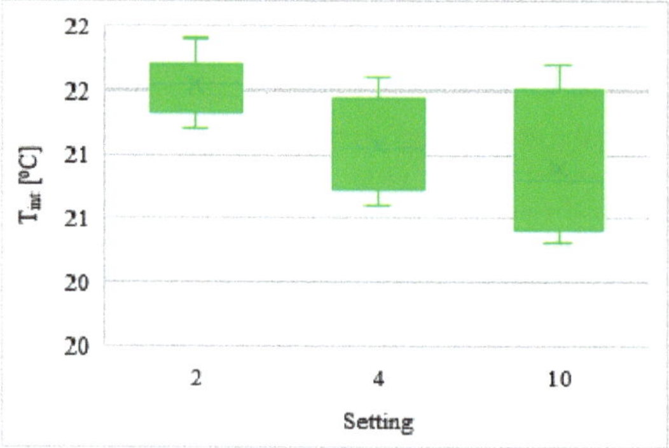

Figure 18. Box plots illustrating the distribution of the *temperature* characteristic in groups defined by *setting* factor levels; T_{int}—temperature, °C.

Figure 19 shows box plots illustrating the distribution of the *temperature* characteristic in groups defined by *location* factor levels. A statistically significant main effect was observed both for *setting* and for *location*. Thus, it is well-grounded to apply the Tukey multiple comparison method.

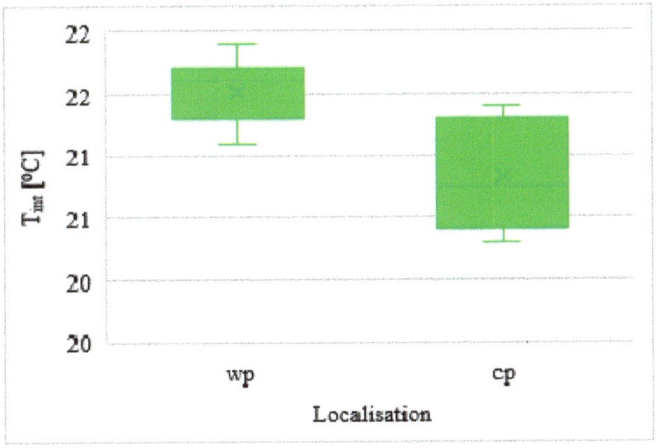

Figure 19. Box plots illustrating the distribution of the *temperature* characteristic in groups defined by *location* factor levels; T_{int}—temperature, °C; wp: workplace; cp: central point.

Table 6 contains the calculation results for the *temperature* characteristic, carried out according to the Tukey method in groups matching the levels of 2, 4, and 10 min of the *setting* factor.

Table 6. The Tukey multiple comparison method tests for the *temperature* characteristic in groups defined on the basis of the *setting* factor levels. No. of Average Values: 3. Least significant difference: 0.12.

Tukey Grouping	Average	N	Setting
A	21.5	12	2
B	21.1	12	4
C	20.9	12	10

Table 6 shows that the highest average *temperature* value should be expected for the 2 min *setting* and the lowest for the 10 min setting.

The data in Table 7 confirm the conclusions derived from Table 6. None of the achieved 95-percent confidence intervals included zero, which means that the differences between average temperature values for each of the pairs were statistically significant. There is a possibility of the quantitative determination of the differences between average temperature values using 95-percent confidence intervals. For example, for the difference in average temperature values in groups matching the 4 min setting and 10 min setting, the extremes were 0.02 and 0.3. Each value within the interval with specified extremes was treated equally as a potential true value of the analyzed difference. Thus, it should be accepted that an average temperature for the 4 min setting may exceed the average temperature for the 2 min setting by either 0.02 or 0.3.

Table 8 contains the calculation results for the *temperature* characteristic, carried out according to the Tukey method in groups matching the following levels: wp (workplace) and cp (central point) of the *location* factor.

Table 7. Simultaneous 95-percent confidence intervals obtained using the Tukey method for the difference in avg. values of *temperature* in groups matching *setting* levels.

Comparison	Difference between Avg. Values	Simultaneous 95-Percent Confidence Intervals	
		Lower Limit	Upper Limit
2–4	0.5	0.3	0.6
4–2	−0.5	−0.6	−0.3
2–10	0.6	0.5	0.8
10–2	−0.6	−0.8	−0.5
4–10	0.2	0.002	0.3
10–4	−0.2	−0.3	−0.002

Table 8. The Tukey multiple comparison method tests for the *temperature* characteristic in groups defined on the basis of the *location* factor levels. No. of Average Values: 2. Least significant difference: 0.096.

Tukey Grouping	Average	N	Setting
A	21.5	18	wp
B	20.8	18	cp

Table 6 shows that the average values of the *temperature* characteristic in the group defined by workplace *location* were significantly higher than those corresponding to the central point location.

The data in Table 9 confirmed the conclusions derived from Table 8. None of the achieved 95-percent confidence intervals included zero, which means that the differences between the average temperature values for each of the pairs were statistically significant. The data allowed for the quantitative determination of the differences between the average temperature values by way of implementing 95-percent confidence intervals. For example, interval extremes for the difference in average temperature values in groups defined by workplace and central point location were 0.6 and 0.8, respectively. Each value within the interval with specified extremes was treated equally as a potential true value of the analyzed difference. Thus, it should be accepted that an average temperature for workplace location may exceed the average temperature for the central point location by either 0.6 or 0.8.

Table 9. Simultaneous 95-percent confidence intervals obtained using the Tukey method for difference in avg. values of *temperature* in groups matching *location* levels.

Comparison	Difference between Avg. Values	Simultaneous 95-Percent Confidence Intervals	
		Lower Limit	Upper Limit
wp–cp	0.7	0.5	0.9
cp–wp	−0.7	−0.9	−0.5

The next step involved carrying out the two-factor ANOVA for the *temperature* characteristic with the following grouping variables: *setting* with values of 2, 4, and 10 min and *outside temperature* with values of −7 °C and −3 °C.

The zero hypothesis stating equality of the average values of the *temperature* characteristic was verified on the basis of all combinations of levels for both equivalent factors. The F statistic was used for this purpose. Table 10 contains the results of the completed calculations used to verify the hypothesis stating the equality of average values of the *temperature* characteristic in groups determined on the basis of both factors.

Table 10. Analysis of variance for the *temperature* characteristic.

Variability	Degrees of Freedom	Sum of the Squares	Mean Square	Value F	Value p
Intergroup	5	2.9	0.6	3.3	0.025
Intragroup	30	5.3	0.2		
Total	35	8.2			

A value *p* obtained for statistic F in the completed test of greater than 0.0001 allows to state that the average values of the *temperature* characteristic did not differ.

Figure 20 demonstrates in box plots the significance of the effect of the interactions between the factors. The distribution of the *temperature* characteristic in groups defined by *setting* and *outside temperature* factors is illustrated in this way.

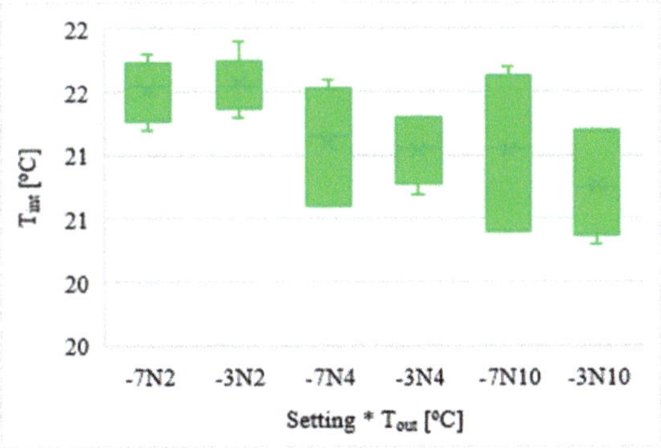

Figure 20. Box plots illustrating the distribution of the *temperature* characteristic in groups defined by pairs of factors: *setting* and *outside temperature*; T_{int}—inside temperature, °C; T_{out}—outside temperature, °C.

Figure 21 shows box plots illustrating the distribution of the *temperature* characteristic in groups defined by the *outside temperature* factor levels.

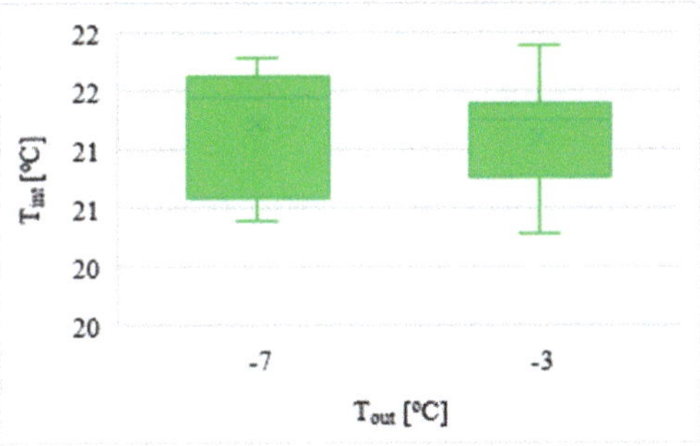

Figure 21. Box plots illustrating the distribution of the *temperature* characteristic in groups defined by *outside temperature* factor levels; T_{int}—temperature, °C; T_{out}—outside temperature, °C

Table 11 contains the calculation results for the *temperature* characteristic, carried out according to the Tukey method in groups matching the levels of −7 °C and −3 °C of the *outside temperature* factor.

Table 11. The Tukey multiple comparison method tests for the *temperature* characteristic in groups defined on the basis of the *outside temperature* factor levels. No. of Average Values: 2. Least significant difference: 0.3.

Tukey Grouping *	Average	N	Setting
A	21.22	18	−7
A	21.12	18	−3

* Average values marked with the same letter do not differ significantly.

Table 11 shows that the average temperature values did not differ significantly.

The two-factor ANOVA for the *humidity* characteristic was carried out in the same way. The grouping variables were: *outside temperature* with the values of −10.5, −10, −9.5, −9, −8.5, −8, −7.5, −7, −6.5, −6, −5.5, −5, −4.5, −4, −3.5, −3, −2.5, −2, −1.5, −1, −0.5, 0, 0.5, 1, 1.5, 2, 2.5, and 3 °C and *location* with the values wp (workplace) and cp (central point).

The zero hypothesis stating equality of the average values of the *humidity* characteristic was verified on the basis of all combinations of levels for both equivalent factors. The F statistic was used for this purpose (the ratio of intergroup variance to intragroup variance). Table 12 contains the results of the completed calculations used to verify the hypothesis stating equality of the average values of the *humidity* characteristic in groups determined on the basis of both factors.

Table 12. Analysis of variance for the humidity characteristic.

Variability	Degrees of Freedom	Sum of the Squares	Mean Square	Value *F*	Value *p*
Intergroup	55	3488.2	63.4	126.9	<0.0001
Intragroup	112	56.0	0.5		
Total	167	3544.2			

A value *p* obtained for statistic F in the completed test of less than 0.0001 allows for the statement that there were at least two groups where the average values of the *humidity* characteristic differed.

Figure 22 demonstrates in box plots the significance of the effect of the interactions between the factors. The distribution of the *humidity* characteristic in groups defined by *outside temperature* and *location* factors is illustrated in this way.

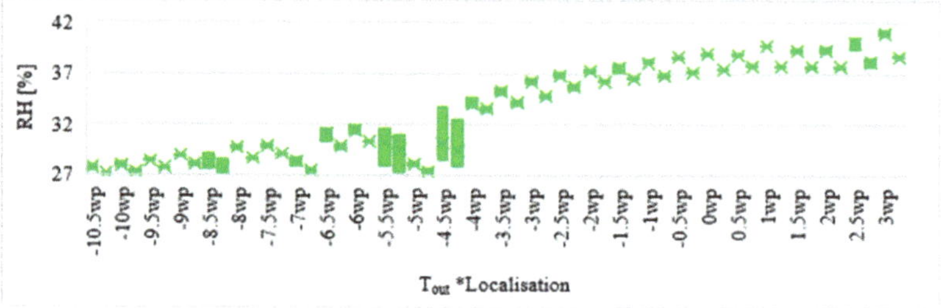

Figure 22. Box plots illustrating the distribution of the *humidity* characteristic in groups defined by pairs of factors: *outside temperature* and *location;* RH_{in}—humidity, %; T_{out}—outside temperature, °C; wp: workplace; cp: central point.

Figure 23 shows box plots illustrating the distribution of the *humidity* characteristic in groups defined by the *outside temperature* factor levels.

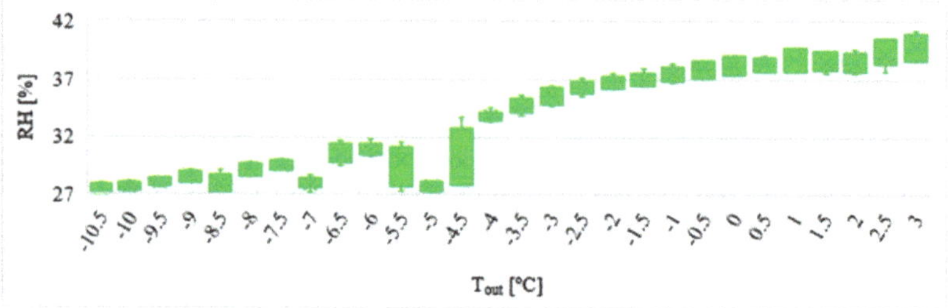

Figure 23. Box plots illustrating the distribution of the *humidity* characteristic in groups defined by *outside temperature* factor levels; RH_{in}—humidity, %; T_{out}—outside temperature, °C.

Table 13 contains the values of the Least Significant Difference LSD and test statistic W for the *humidity* characteristic, carried out according to the Tukey method in groups matching the levels of −10.5, −10, −9.5, −9, −8.5, −8, −7.5, −7, −6.5, −6, −5.5, −5, −4.5, −4, −3.5, −3, −2.5, −2, −1.5, −1, −0.5, 0, 0.5, 1, 1.5, 2, 2.5, and 3 °C of the *outside temperature* factor.

Table 13. The Tukey multiple comparison method tests for the *humidity* characteristic in groups defined on the basis of the *outside temperature* factor levels.

No. of Average Values	28
Least Significant Difference	0.15
Test Statistic W	1.18

The tests of multiple comparisons carried out using the Tukey method for the *humidity* characteristic in groups defined by the outside temperature showed that the highest average humidity value should be expected for the outside temperature of 3 °C, and the lowest for the outside temperature of −10.5 °C.

Figure 24 shows box plots illustrating the distribution of the *humidity* characteristic in groups defined by the *location* factor levels.

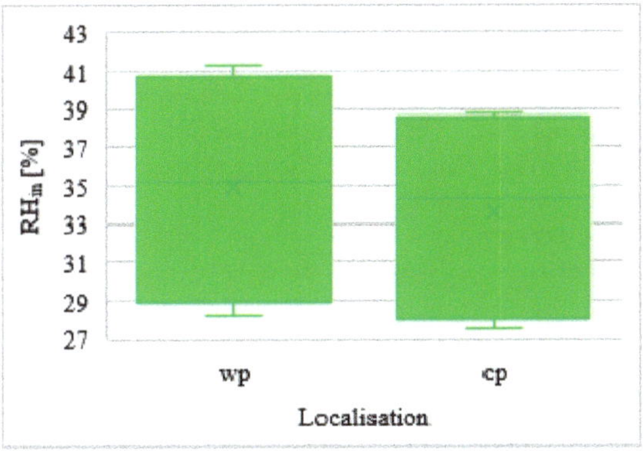

Figure 24. Box plots illustrating the distribution of the *humidity* characteristic in groups defined by the *location* factor levels; RH_{in}—humidity, %; wp: workplace; cp: central point.

Table 14 contains the calculation results for the *humidity* characteristic, carried out according to the Tukey method in groups matching the workplace and central point levels of the *location* factor.

Table 14. The Tukey multiple comparison method tests for the *humidity* characteristic in groups defined on the basis of the *location* factor levels. No. of Average Values: 2. Least significant difference: 0.08.

Tukey Grouping	Average	N	Setting
A	34.9	42	wp
B	33.6	42	cp

Table 14 shows that the average values of the *humidity* characteristic in the group defined by the workplace *location* were significantly higher than those corresponding to the central point *location*.

4. Conclusions

The interior microclimate is extremely important for the health and well-being of people staying in rooms. Sick building syndrome is a current problem that many building administrators and users must cope with, and most often results from an insufficient air exchange, occurring as a consequence of the excessive sealing of buildings. By and large, a great majority of existing buildings are ventilated naturally. Thermal modernization works are usually limited to the thermal insulation of building cladding and providing airtight window joinery. In most cases, there is no possibility of installing mechanical ventilation systems. In these cases, decentralized façade units may be the right solution for occupants to improve the indoor microclimate. Completed analysis of the patented solution has proven that, in spite of the lack of heat recovery exchanger and air heater, the unit does not reduce the inside air temperature below the comfort level while replacing used air with fresh air. Throughout the period of measurements, temperature values ranged within 20–22 °C. Moreover, the PMV value calculated on the basis of measurements showed that in the workplace, category B was maintained in the area of the head, abdomen, and feet, and the central point of the room was in category C at the end of the cycle (2 min). In the long cycle (10 min), it belonged to category C for almost the entire duration of the airflow (at all parts of the body). However, it should be mentioned that there is a risk of a local sensation of discomfort (draught) in the case where a user stands in the axis of the air stream and the air supply/exhaust cycle is long. In this case, the DR index at a distance of 70 cm from the supply/exhaust grate at the level of abdomen may be as high as 64%. It is recommended to use heat recovery from exhaust air and possibly an electric heater to warm up the air in order to eliminate the risk of negative air movement impact and the sensation of discomfort. Further studies will focus on the search for an optimal way to recover heat for decentralized ventilation units.

Air humidity analysis has proven that the value of this parameter value was too low and ranged within 27 to 43%. This indicates the need to find a way to humidify air in decentralized façade units.

The analyses of both temperature and humidity have proven that the values of inside air temperature and humidity are not affected by the temperature and humidity of outside air. In this case, it is important that negative pressure generated during the exhaust cycle induces an inflow of warm and dry air from an adjacent room.

The impact of using the decentralized façade unit on inside air parameters was analyzed for each of the three durations of air supply/exhaust cycle (2 min, 4 min, 10 min). In each of these cases, no temperature drop in the room was observed, and the air humidity was too low. Research results obtained during the experiment were evaluated from the statistical point of view. Completed statistical analysis proved that the average temperature values did not differ significantly for the outside temperature factor. On the other hand, in the case of the air supply/exhaust cycle duration setting, the average inside temperature was the highest for the shortest cycle and the lowest for the longest cycle.

In conclusion, it is necessary to carry out further tests of the decentralized façade units that would be used as an efficient way to improve the interior microclimate. However, it is necessary to find methods for heat recovery and air humidification.

5. Patents

The article presents the test results of patent-protected equipment: Zender-Świercz E., Piotrowski J. *Room ventilation unit* (2017). Patent no. PL 228624 B1.

Funding: This research was funded by the program of the Minister of Science and Higher Education under the name: "Regional Initiative of Excellence" in 2019–2022 project number 025/RID/2018/19, financing amount PLN 12,000,000.

Conflicts of Interest: The author declares no conflict of interest.

References

1. Apte, M.G.; Fisk, W.J.; Daisey, J.M. Association between indoor CO_2 concentration and sick building syndrome symptoms in U.S. office buildings:an analysis of the 1994—1996 BASE study data. *Indoor Air* **2000**, *10*, 246–257. [CrossRef] [PubMed]
2. Apte, M.G.; Fisk, W.J.; Daisey, J.M. Indoor carbon dioxide concentrations and SBS in office workers. *Proc. Healthy Build.* **2000**, *1*, 133–138.

3. Daisey, J.M.; Angell, W.J.; Apte, M. Indoor air quality, ventilation and health symptoms in schools: An analysis of existing information. *Indoor Air* **2003**, *13*, 53–64. [CrossRef] [PubMed]
4. Haverinen-Shaughnessy, U.; Moschandreas, D.J.; Shaughnessy, R.J. Association between substandard classroom ventilation rates and students academic achievement. *Indoor Air* **2011**, *21*, 121–131. [CrossRef] [PubMed]
5. Huttunen, K. Indoor Air Pollution. In *Clinical Handbook of Air Pollution—Retated Diseases*; Capello, F., Gaddi, A.V., Eds.; Springer: Modena, Italy, 2018; pp. 107–114. [CrossRef]
6. Mendell, M.J.; Heath, G.A. Do indoor pollutants and thermal conditions in school influence student performance? A critical review of the literature. *Indoor Air* **2005**, *15*, 27–52. [CrossRef] [PubMed]
7. Seppanen, O.A.; Fisk, W.J. Effects of temperature and outdoor air supply rate on the performance of call center operators in the tropics. *Indoor Air* **2004**, *7*, 102–118. [CrossRef] [PubMed]
8. Seppanen, O.A.; Fisk, W.J.; Mendel, M.J. Association of ventilation rates and CO_2 concentrations with health and other responses in commercial and industrial buildings. *Indoor Air* **1999**, *9*, 226–252. [CrossRef]
9. Sowa, J. Jakość powietrza we wnętrzach jako istoty element pływający na komfort pracy. *Cyrkulacje* **2017**, *37*, 32–33.
10. Telejko, M.; Zender-Świercz, E. An attempt to improve air quality in primary schools. 10th International Conference. *Environ. Eng.* **2017**. [CrossRef]
11. Zender-Świercz, E. Improving the indoor air quality using the Indyvidual Air Supply System. *Int. J. Environ. Sci. Technol.* **2018**, *15*, 689–696. [CrossRef]
12. Zender-Świercz, E.; Telejko, M. The impact of insulation building on the work of ventilation. *Procedia Eng.* **2016**, *161*, 1731–1737. [CrossRef]
13. Górny, R.L. *Submikronowe Cząstki Grzybów i Bakterii—Nowe Zagrożenie Środowiska Wnętrz*; Wydawnictwa Politechniki Warszawskiej: Warsaw, Poland, 2005; pp. 25–40.
14. Fisk, W.J.; Mirer, A.G.; Mendell, M.J. Quantitative relationship of sick building syndrome symptoms with ventilation rates. *Indoor Air* **2009**, *19*, 159–165. [CrossRef] [PubMed]
15. Muchič, S.; Butala, V. The influence of indoor environment in office building on their occupants: Expected—Unexpected. *Build. Environ.* **2004**, *39*, 289–296. [CrossRef]
16. Runeson, R.; Wahlstedt, K.; Wieslander, G.; Norbäck, D. Personal and psychosocial factors and symptoms compatible with sick building syndrome in the Swedish workforce. *Indoor Air* **2006**, *16*, 445–453. [CrossRef] [PubMed]
17. Brasche, S.; Bullinger, M.; Morfeld, M.; Gebhardt, H.J.; Bischof, W. Why do Women Suffer from Sick Building Syndrome more often than Men?—Subjective Higher Sensitivity versus Objective Causes. *Indoor Air* **2001**, *11*, 217–222. [CrossRef] [PubMed]
18. Karjalainen, S. Gender differences in thermal comfort and use of thermostats in everyday thermal environments. *Build. Environ.* **2007**, *42*, 1594–1603. [CrossRef]
19. Karjalainen, S. Thermal comfort and gender: A literature review. *Indoor Air* **2012**, *22*, 96–109. [CrossRef]
20. Winarti, M.; Basuki, B.; Hamid, A. Air movement, gender and risk of sick building headache among employees in a Jakarta office. *Med. J. Indones.* **2003**, *12*, 171–177. [CrossRef]
21. Lan, L.; Wargocki, P.; Lian, Z. Quantitative measurement of productivity loss due to thermal discomfort. *Energy Build.* **2011**, *43*, 1057–1062. [CrossRef]
22. Klavina, A.; Proskurina, J.; Rodins, V.; Martinsone, I. Carbon dioxide as indoor air quality indicator in renovated schools in Latvia. In Proceedings of the Indoor Air 2016 The 14th International Conference of Indoor Air Quality and Climate, Ghent, Belgium, 3–8 July 2016.
23. Roelofsen, P. The impact of office environments on employee performance:the design of the workplace as strategy for productivity enhancement. *J. Facil. Manag.* **2002**, *1*, 247–264. [CrossRef]
24. Johnson, D.L.; Lynch, R.A.; Floyd, E.L.; Wang, J.; Bartels, J.N. Indoor air quality in classrooms: Environmental measures and effective ventilation rate modeling in urban elementary schools. *Build. Environ.* **2018**. [CrossRef]
25. Vimalanathan, K.; Babu, T.R. The effect of indoor office environment on the work performance, health and welbeing of office workers. *J. Environ. Health Sci.* **2014**, *12*, 113. [CrossRef] [PubMed]
26. Mijakowski, M. *Wilgotność Powietrza w Relacjach Człowiek, Środowisko Wewnętrzne, Architektura*; Wydawnictwa Politechniki Warszawskiej: Warsaw, Poland, 2005; pp. 105–121.

27. Polish Committee for Standardization. *PN EN 13788:2013-05 Hygrothermal Performance of Building Components and Building Elements—Internal Surface Temperature to Avoid Critical Surface Humidity and Interstitial Condensation—Calculation Methods*; Polish Committee for Standardization: Warszawa, Poland, 2016.
28. Pogorzelski, J.A. *Zagadnienia Cieplno—Wilgotnościowe Przegród Budowlanych*; Budownictwo ogólne, P., Ed.; Arkady: Warsaw, Poland, 2005.
29. Kisilewicz, T. O związkach między szczelnością budynków, a mikroklimatem, komfortem wewnętrznym i zużyciem energii w budynkach niskoenergetycznych. *Napędy Sterow.* **2014**, *12*, 94–97.
30. Lazovic, I.; Stevanović, Z.M.; Jovašević-Stojanović, M.; Živković, M.M.; Banjac, M. Impact of CO_2 concentration on indoor air quality and correlation with relative humidity and indoor air temperature in school building in Serbia. *Therm. Sci.* **2015**, *20*, 173. [CrossRef]
31. Nomura, M.; Hiyama, K. A review: Natural ventilation performance of office buildings in Japan. *Renew. Sustain. Energy Rev.* **2017**, *74*, 746–754. [CrossRef]
32. Fanger, P.O.; Popiołek, Z.; Wargocki, P. *Środowisko Wewnętrzne. Wpływ na Zdrowie, Komfort i Wydajność Pracy*; Wydawnictwo Politechniki Śląskiej: Gliwice, Poland, 2003.
33. Fanger, P.O.; Melikov, A.K.; Hanzawa, H.; Ring, J. Air turbulence and sensation of draught. *Energy Build.* **1988**, *12*, 21–39. [CrossRef]
34. Toftum, J.; Zhou, G.; Melikov, A.K. Effect of Airflow Direction on Human Perception of Draught. Available online: https://pdfs.semanticscholar.org/3a9b/c78141659022d3e207879b65a240c9820ea4.pdf (accessed on 20 May 2020).
35. Coydon, F.; Herkel, S.; Kuber, T.; Pfafferott, J.; Himmelsbach, S. Energy performance of façade integrated decentralised ventilation systems. *Energy Build.* **2015**, *107*, 172–180. [CrossRef]
36. Merzkirch, A.; Mass, S.; Scholzen, F.; Waldmann, D. Primary energy used in centralised and decentralised ventilation systems measured in field tests in residential buildings. *Int. J. Vent.* **2019**, *18*, 19–27. [CrossRef]
37. Dermentzis, G.; Ochs, F.; Siegele, D.; Feist, W. Renovation with an innovative compact heating and ventilation system integrated into the façade—An in-situ monitoring case study. *Energy Build.* **2018**, *165*, 451–463. [CrossRef]
38. Gruner, M.; Haase, M. The Potential of Façade-Integrated Ventilation Systems in Nordic Climate. In *Advanced Decentralised Ventilation Systems as Sustainable Alternative to Conventional Systems*; NTNU: Trondheim, Norway, 2012.
39. Energy Performance of Buildings. *Ventilation for Buildings. Indoor Environmental Input Parameters for Design and Assessment of Energy Performance of Buildings Addressing Indoor Air Quality, Thermal Environment, Lighting and Acoustics. Module M1-6*; PN EN 16798-1:2019-06; Polish Committee for Standardization: Warsaw, Poland, 2019.
40. *Indoor Environmental Input Parameters for Design and Assessment of Energy Performance of Buildings Addressing Indoor Air Quality, Thermal Environment, Lighting and Acoustics*; PN EN 15251: 2012; Polish Committee for Standardization: Warsaw, Poland, 2012.
41. Mikola, A.; Simson, R.; Kurnitski, J. The Impact of Air Pressure Conditions on the Performance of Single Room Ventilation Units in Multi-Story Buildings. *Energies* **2019**, *12*, 2633. [CrossRef]
42. Zemitis, J.; Bogdanovics, R. Heat recovery efficiency of local decentralized ventilation devices. *Mag. Civ. Eng.* **2020**, *94*, 120–128. [CrossRef]
43. *Ergonomics of the Thermal Environment—Analytical Determination and Interpretation of Thermal Comfort Using Calculation of the PMV and PPD Indices and Local Thermal Comfort Criteria*; PN EN 7730; Polish Committee for Standardization: Warsaw, Poland, 2006.
44. Catalina, T.; Istrate, M.A.; Damian, A.; Vartires, A.; Dicu, T.; Cucoş, A. Indoor air quality assessment in a classroom using a heat recovery ventilation unit. *Rom. J. Phys.* **2019**, *64*, 9–10.
45. *Ventilation for Acceptable Indoor Air Quality*; ASHRAE-ANSI-ASHRAE Standard 62.1-2016; ASHRAE: Atlanta, GA, USA, 2016.

atmosphere

MDPI

Article

Efficacy of Radiant Catalytic Ionization in Reduction of *Enterococcus* spp., *Clostridioides difficile* and *Staphylococcus aureus* in Indoor Air

Krzysztof Skowron [1,*], Katarzyna Grudlewska-Buda [1], Sylwia Kożuszko [1], Natalia Wiktorczyk [1], Karolina Jadwiga Skowron [2], Agnieszka Mikucka [1], Zuzanna Bernaciak [1] and Eugenia Gospodarek-Komkowska [1]

1 Department of Microbiology, Nicolaus Copernicus University in Toruń, Ludwik Rydygier Collegium Medicum, 9 M. Skłodowskiej-Curie Street, 85-094 Bydgoszcz, Poland; katinkag@gazeta.pl (K.G.-B.); kozuszko@cm.umk.pl (S.K.); natalia12127@gmail.com (N.W.); a.mikucka@cm.umk.pl (A.M.); zuza.bernaciak@gmail.com (Z.B.); gospodareke@cm.umk.pl (E.G.-K.)

2 Institute of Telecommunications and Computer Science, UTP University of Science and Technology, Al. prof. S. Kaliskiego 7, 85-796 Bydgoszcz, Poland; kj.skowron@wp.pl

* Correspondence: skowron238@wp.pl; Tel.: +48-(52)-585-38-38

Received: 16 June 2020; Accepted: 17 July 2020; Published: 20 July 2020

check for updates

Abstract: (1) Background: An aerogenic way is one of main rout of spreading microorganisms (including antibiotic resistant), that cause healthcare-associated infections. The source of microorganisms in the air can be patients, personnel, visitors, outdoor air, hospital surfaces and equipment, and even sink drains. (2) Methods: The standardized suspensions (0.5 McFarland) of the examined strains (*Enterococcus* spp., *Clostridioides difficile, Staphylococcus aureus*) were nebulized in sterile chamber. Then the Induct 750 (ActivTek) device, generating RCI (radiant catalytic ionization) phenomenon, was used for 20 min. Next, the number of bacteria in the air was calculated using collision method. The percentage of reduction coefficient (R) was calculated. (3) Results: In case of enterococci, the R value was >90% and there are no statistically significant differences among tested strains. For *C. difficile* strains the R value range from 64–95%. The R value calculated for hypervirulent, antibiotic resistant CDI PCR 27 strain was statistically significantly lower than for other examined strains. For *S. aureus* non-MRSA the R value was 99.87% and for *S. aurues* MRSA the R value was 95.61%. (4) Conclusions: The obtained results indicate that the use of RCI may contribute to reducing the occurrence of dangerous pathogens in the air, and perhaps transmission and persistence in the hospital buildings environment.

Keywords: radiant catalytic ionization; *Enterococcus* spp.; *Clostridioides difficile*; *Staphylococcus aureus*; MRSA; indoor air

1. Introduction

Healthcare-associated infections (HAIs) are a very serious medical problem. HAIs pose a threat to hospitalized patients. They mainly affect person with a weak immune system. Hospital infections most often affect people in intensive care units. They are usually caused by multi-resistant bacteria with high spreading potential. One of the directions of action is striving to limit patients' contact with pathogenic microorganisms in the air. The problem of nosocomial infections can be minimized through appropriate control and monitoring systems [1].

Many actions are taken to prevent spread of microorganism. These activities include: antibiotic prevention and therapies, cleaning and disinfection of the surface, hygiene of the hands and clothing of the staff, separation of special areas, isolation of patients with diarrhea, etc., [1].

However, one of the main ways of spreading microorganisms that cause HAI—an aerogenic path—is often overlooked. Unfortunately, for many years, the transmission of pathogenic microorganisms by air was not considered a serious health risk [2]. However, there is a lot of evidence that suggests that both Gram-negative and Gram-positive bacteria are often spread by air in the hospital environment [1]. The hospital environment is a very dynamic environment from the microbiological point of view. The composition of bioaerosol generated in hospital rooms is usually very diverse. The source of microorganisms present in the air can be patients, personnel, visitors, outdoor air, hospital surfaces and equipment, and even sink drains [3,4]. Factors affecting the presence of microbes in hospital air include seasons, weather conditions (e.g., temperature, humidity), efficient ventilation system, humidity, number of patients and guests, as well as activities such as how often the door is opened or staff and guests move [5,6]. Microorganisms can get into the air during medical treatments and even during simple maintenance activities, such as changes in bedding or clothing [7]. It was also shown that contaminated air-conditioning devices were the source of *P. aeruginosa* infection [1]. It was shown that in the environment of patients infected with methicillin-resistant *Staphylococcus aureus* (MRSA), 4.7 CFU m^3 of MRSA, and during bed turn down the number of bacteria increased up to 116 CFU m^3 [7]. The problem of bioaerosol formation by Gram-negative bacteria is particularly dangerous in relation to medical equipment, e.g., humidifiers, nebulizers, respirators, which is associated with respiratory infections [1]. The main route of infectious bioaerosol spread in the hospital are ventilation systems. There are two main types of ventilation systems—natural and mechanical [8], which choice depends on the type of room. Mechanical fans can be installed directly in windows or walls or installed in air ducts to supply air to or extract air from the room [9,10]. Through ventilation system, pathogenic microorganisms from one patient can spread to other rooms or even other floors of the building, and can also sediment on various surfaces in other rooms, causing their contamination [9]. Proper maintenance of ventilation systems can help to reduce infection [10].

Among the microorganisms spreading through the aerogenic pathway in hospitals, multi-drug resistant (MDR) enterococci, *C. difficile* and MRSA are important.

Enterococcus spp. are a natural microbiota of the digestive tract of humans and animals. *Enterococcus spp.* may be the etiological factor of various forms of clinical infections, especially urinary tract, endocarditis, peritonitis, and burn wound infections. Most nosocomial infections are caused by biofilm forming bacteria, which allows them to survive in the urinary tract, avoiding the host's immune response. Increasingly, MDR strains of *Enterococcus* spp. are isolated in the hospital environment. Currently, enterococci are classified as alarm pathogens. They are among the most dangerous multi-drug resistant pathogens, called the ESKAPE acronym (*Enterococcus faecium*, *Staphylococcus aureus*, *Klebsiella pneumoniae*, *Acinetobacter baumannii*, *Pseudomonas aeruginosa*, *Enterobacter* spp.), responsible for infections associated with healthcare (HAIs) [11].

The majority of enterococcal infections are endogenous, however, exogenous infections are more frequently found in hospitalized patients and result from transmission of strains from other patients or the hospital environment. The primary mode of spread from patient-to-patient occurs through the hands of healthcare workers [12]. In recent decades, an increase in isolation of *Enterococcus* spp. resistant to ampicillin and vancomycin from the hospital environment was noticed. This tendency applies in particular *Enterococcus faecium* strains. This applies mainly to the acquisition of vancomycin resistance among these strains (Vancomycin Resistant Enterococcus, VRE) [11]. A frequent among enterococci is the simultaneous occurrence of several mechanisms of resistance to antibiotics from different chemical groups [13].

C. difficile is currently one of the most important pathogens responsible for antibiotic-associated diarrhea and *pseudomembranous colitis*, mainly in hospital patients, but increasingly also in non-hospital patients, including persons without risk factors [14]. Pathogenic *C. difficile* strains produce toxin A (TcdA, encoded by the *tcdA* gene) and/or toxin B (TcdB, encoded by the *tcdB* gene). Toxins cause, among others, destruction of the cytoskeleton, apoptosis of epithelial cells, induction of proinflammatory cytokine production, recruitment of inflammatory cells, contributing to the destruction of intercellular connections, which, with the participation of hydrolytic enzymes, leads to the development of colitis, pseudomembrane, and diarrhea [14,15]. Since the emergence of hypervirulent ribotype PCR 027 in Europe, there has been an increase in *C. difficile* infection (CDI) cases, mortality, and further evolution of strains to increase virulence, the possibility of spreading in the environment and resistance to antibiotics [15]. Resistance to moxifloxacin may be a marker of increased virulence of *C. difficile* strains [16]. Roberts et al. [17] and Best et al. [18] demonstrated that *C. difficile* can easily spread in the hospital environment through aerogenic pathways. Spores play a major role in the spread and maintenance of *C. difficile* strains in the hospital environment [19]. Spores are formed after 15 min of exposure of vegetative forms to oxygen, they are resistant to many hygienization and disinfection procedures [20]. Evidence for this is provided by the frequent isolation of *C. difficile* spores from ventilation ducts in hospitals and high horizontal surfaces [21]. The mean spore length is 1–1.5 mm and the mean diameter is 0.5–0.7 μm, although there is documented significant variation in individual sizes of spores both within and between strains. Fallout time of *C. difficile* spores in a still room from 1 m height range from 2.1 to 13.9 h [22]. Furthermore, it was suggested that aerial dissemination could play a role in the persistence of *C. difficile* in hospitals [19].

S. aureus is an opportunistic human pathogen [23,24], which can cause, among others, wound infections, pneumonia in immunocompromised individuals, chest abscess and bacteraemia [25]. *S. aureus* is listed as one of the most common pathogens responsible for nosocomial infections [23]. About a third of the population is carriers of *S. aureus*. It usually colonizes wet areas, such as armpits, groin, and nose, although it can also be found on other parts of the body, for example on the hands [23]. In contrast, MRSA (Methicillin-resistant *Staphylococcus aureus*) strains are of particular concern because of their resistance to β-lactam antibiotics, which makes treatment more difficult [25]. This pathogen is currently responsible for about 61% of staphylococcal infections [25]. The basic mode of transmission of MRSA strains within the hospital are temporarily colonized hands of hospital staff. In addition, it is believed that MRSA in the form of bioaerosol can pollute the air. Although the transmission of MRSA in the air is generally considered less frequent than the transmission by direct contact, it is considered that air is an important factor to be considered in hospital wards [26]. Both *S. aureus* and MRSA in the air are present in the form of particles with an aerodynamic diameter that can accumulate in the human upper respiratory tract, primary, secondary, and final bronchi and alveoli. The spherical cells of *S. aureus* are up to maximal 1 μm in diameter [23–26].

Therefore, it is important to look for the effective methods to maintain microbiological purity of the air and ventilation systems. One of them is radiant catalytic ionization (RCI). RCI [27] is an active method of air and surface cleaning. The RCI cell consists of matrices of elongated polycarbonate components, arranged in a parallel orientation resembling a honeycomb. A coating of matrices comprises a grouping of the materials: titanium dioxide, rhodium, silver, and copper. On the opposite site a broad-spectrum UV light source is located. The UV lamp utilizes argon gas with mercury and carbide filaments with a spectrum of 100 and 367 nm [28,29]. It works by creating a proper wavelength and using the photo-oxidation effect with the participation of UV light and appropriate photocatalysers such as TiO_2, which are placed in the hydrophilic coverage of the RCI chamber [28]. The result is generation of biocidal reactive oxygen species (ROS), hydroxyl radicals ($OH^{\bullet}$), superoxide radicals ($O_2^{-\bullet}$), hydro-peroxyl radical ($HO_2^{\bullet}$), and hydrogen peroxide (H_2O_2) [28,29]. The manufacturer declares that the total number of generated ions is about 5.0×10^5 ions cm^{-3} of air. In addition, in photocatalytic oxidation also other secondary impurities aldehydes: acetaldehyde and formaldehyde are produced. Also aldehydes have harmful health effects [30,31]. Photocatalysis has been found to not only effectively eliminate Gram-positive and Gram-negative bacteria, spores, viruses, fungi, and protozoa but also inactivate prions and bacterial toxins [32]. Gram-positive bacteria have been shown to be more resistant to photocatalytic disinfection than Gram-negative [28]. Their action is related to the oxidation of coenzyme A molecules, which inhibits the respiratory pathway, oxidation of unsaturated phospholipids, interactions with extracellular polymeric substances (EPS), and causes the accumulation of DNA and RNA damage in the bacterial cell [32–34]. Despite the ozone generation during the operation of the device, it has been shown that it is not a main bactericidal agent, because at the time of air exchange its level does not exceed 0.05 ppm [28,33,35]. It is important that WHO Air Quality Quidelines 2005 gives for ozone 8-h mean limit of 100 μg/m^3. WHO points out that sensitive individual may have health effects also in lower concentrations than the limit. It is very important that the producer of the equipment not only says, but also offers some reliably tested proofs about the measured levels of the produced ozone. According to USA EPA ozone generators have many harmful health effects [36]. In case of tested RCI device, its producer declares ozone production at a level below 0.04 ppm [35]. Currently, new version of RCI devices does not generate ozone.

The aim of the study is to assess the efficiency of RCI in eliminating enterococci resistant to selected antibiotics in the air compared to the antibiotic-susceptible strain, antibiotic-resistant, toxinogenic *C. difficile* in comparison with the non-toxinogenic, antibiotic-susceptible strain and elimination of *S. aureus* non-MRSA and MRSA strain.

2. Materials and Methods

2.1. Materials

The research material consisted of three *Enterococcus* spp. standard strains, three *C. difficile* strains isolated, and two *S. aureus* strains from a clinical specimen from the collection of the Department of Microbiology, Ludwik Rydygier Collegium Medicum. in Bydgoszcz, Nicolaus Copernicus University in Toruń:

Enterococcus faecalis PCM 1861, isolated from clinical material, susceptible to antibiotics.

Enterococcus faecalis ATCC 51299, isolated from a peritoneal fluid sample from a patient from Saint Louis, Missouri, USA, resistant to vancomycin, gentamicin, streptomycin, and erythromycin, with confirmed presence of genes: *vanB* i *ant(6)-I acc(6′) aph(2′′′′)*.

Enterococcus faecium ATCC 51559, isolated from a patient from Brooklyn, New York, USA, resistant to vancomycin, teicoplanin, ampicillin, gentamycin, ciprofloxacin, and rifampicin, with confirmed presence of *vanA* gene.

C. difficile non-toxigenic strain (CDI tox(−)).

C. difficile strain producing A, B, and binary toxins and resistant to moxifloxacin (CDI MXF-R/tox A/B/bin(+)).

C. difficile PCR-ribotype 027 strain (CDI PCR 027).

S. aureus MRSA isolated from wound infection.

S. aureus non-MRSA isolated from wound infection.

All strains were plated on Columbia Agar with 5% sheep blood (Becton-Dickinson) and incubated at 37 °C for 24 h. After this time, the grown strains were transfer on the same type of medium, and the grown colonies were used in the next stages of the study. *C. difficile* was incubated under anaerobic conditions (Genbag anaer atmosphere generator (bioMérieux) at 37 °C for 48 h.

2.2. RCI Efficiently

For the purpose of the study, standardized suspensions of the examined strains were prepared from fresh culture in physiological saline (Polpharma) with an optical density of 0.5 McFarland standard using a densitometer (DEN-1B, Biosan). The bacterial concentration in the suspension was respectively for *Enterococcus* spp. 2.38×10^8 CFU cm^{-3} ($\pm 5.26 \times 10^7$); *C. difficile* 7.25×10^7 ($\pm 1.66 \times 10^7$) CFU cm^{-3}; *S. aureus* 1.72×10^8 ($\pm 4.17 \times 10^7$) CFU cm^{-3}. In case of *C. difficile*, the suspensions of vegetative cells of the tested strains were used. However, further handling with suspension lasting about 50 min was not conducted in anaerobic conditions, which could lead to the formation of spores. As a result, the spontaneously arose mixtures of vegetative forms and spores of *C. difficile* were RCI treated during the experiment. This reflected the actual conditions for the spread of *C. difficile* in hospitals.

Then, 4 mL of each suspension was placed individually in a sterile nebulizer chamber of the MONSUN MP1 (Medbryt) pneumatic inhaler. Nebulization was carried out until the inhaler chamber was completely emptied (about 15 min). The capacity of the nebulizer compressor is 15.5 L/min and the maximal aerosol capacity is 0.48 mL/min with a particle diameter of 1.4–2.4 μm.

The nebulizer chamber was placed in the test room, which was a hermetic chamber, with a volume of 1.4 m^3 made of steel plates. The chamber is closed with a front wall made of polycarbonate placed in a metal frame. This wall is screwed and closed with side closures. All connections are sealed. The hermetic test was carried out using colored smoke generated by Björnax smoke candles. Before each subsequent nebulization, the walls of the chamber were disinfected chemically with an agent intended for disinfection of solid surfaces, and the air contained in it was subjected to UV-C lamp Philips TUV 36W/G36 T8 for 20 min. After this time, the chamber was opened for about 20 min to remove accumulated ozone. During ventilation the chamber, in the test room the airflow UV-C lamp, which does not generate ozone, was turning on. Moreover, the air and surfaces in the test room were subjected to UV-C radiation for 2 h, before the start the experiment. Before commencing nebulization a control assessment of microbiological purity of the air was carried out in order to check the so-called microbiological background level. A detailed experimental design is shown in Figure 1, and the appearance of research set is presented in Figure 2. Each experiment was conducted in triplicate for each strains.

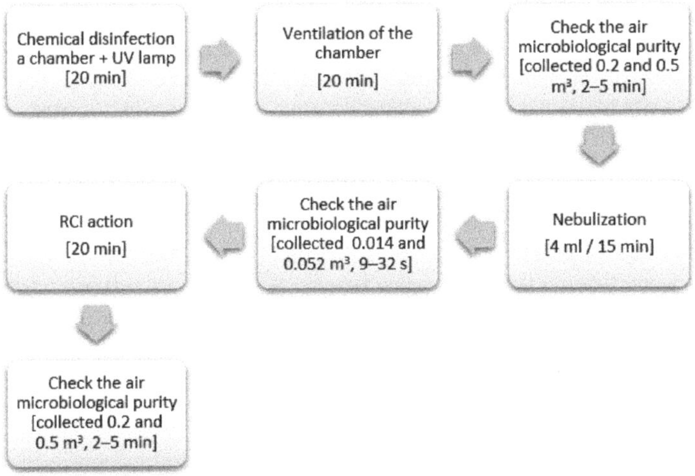

Figure 1. Detailed experimental design according [37].

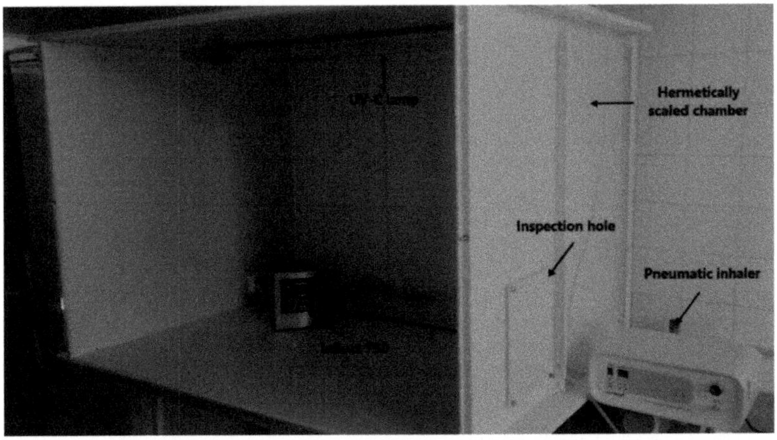

Figure 2. Appearance of research set according [37].

The air samples were sampled using the collision method with MAS-100 Eco (Merck) device. The nominal air flow through the sampler head is 100 L/min. In order to assess the microbiological purity of the air after using Philips TUV 36W/G36 T8 UV-C lamps and Induct 750 devices, 0.2 and 0.5 m^3 were taken. However, in order to assess the level of bacterial contamination in the chamber after nebulization of the bacterial suspension, 0.01 and 0.05 m^3 were sampled. *Enterococcus* spp. bacteria were cultured on Enterococcosel Agar (Becton-Dickinson) at 35 °C for 24 h. *C. difficile* were grown on chromID® *C. difficile* (bioMérieux) under anaerobic conditions generated with Genbag anaer atmosphere generator (bioMérieux) at 37 °C for 48 h. *S. aureus* strains were cultured on mannitol salt agar (Becton Dickinson). The colonies growing on the agar were counted and converted into colony forming units (CFU) m^{-3} of air. Effectiveness was expressed by giving the number of CFU before and after using the Induct 750, and calculating the percentage reduction (R [%]) according to the formula:

$$R_{RCI}[\%] = \frac{A - B}{A} \times 100 \quad (1)$$

where: A—the initial number of microorganisms [CFU m^{-3}], B—the number of microorganisms after using the device [CFU m^{-3}].

The positive control in the study was suspensions of the microorganisms tested, which were nebulized and not exposed to RCI. Samples in the volume of 0.2 and 0.5 m^3 were taken after 20 min. In this way, spontaneous precipitate overtime was evaluated. Precipitate factor was expressed by giving the number of CFU directly after neubulization and 20 min after nebulization, and calculating the percentage reduction $R_{witout\ RCI}$ [%] according to the formula presented above, where B was the number of microorganisms after 20 min from nebulization without RCI action [CFU m^{-3}].

2.3. Experimental Environment Conditions

In addition, negative ion concentration was measured in the chamber air before and after the RCI technology usage. The measurement was made using air negative ion measuring instrument KT-401 AIR (VKTECH)—measurement range 10^4–10^6 ions cm^{-3}. The air temperature and humidity in the chamber was also measured using the thermo-hygrometer LB-710AL (Lab-El).

2.4. Statistical Analysis

The obtained results were subjected to statistical analysis in the STATISTICA 13.0 PL (TIBCO Software, Palo Alto Networks, Inc., Santa Clara, CA, USA). The significance of differences between the values of R coefficients calculated for the strains of a given species was checked based on Tukey's test at the significance level of 0.05.

3. Results

3.1. Experimental Environment Coditions

The experimental environment conditions are presented in Table 1.

Table 1. Basic experimental environment conditions.

Parameter	RCI Technology Usage	
	Before	**After**
Negative ions concentration [ion cm^{-3}]	<1.0 × 10^4	7.2 × 10^5 (±0.7 × 10^5)
Temperature [°C]	25.3 (±0.4)	24.8 (±0.2)
Relative humidity [%]	50.4 (±1.1)	49.2 (±0.8)

3.2. Changes in the Number of *Enterococcus* spp. in the Air

The obtained results showed some fluctuations of the CFU number of tested enterococci present in the air after nebulization of suspensions (Table 2). For this reason, it was decided to introduce an absolute reduction measure in the form of R [%].

After the nebulization, it was found that the tested strains of *Enterococcus* spp. in a similar number spread in the form of an aerosol (Table 2).

The use of RCI resulted in a significant decrease in the CFU number both *E. faecalis* and *E. faecium* strains in the air. CFU number of all tested strains decreased by over 90%. The highest decrease was observed in the *E. faecalis* PCM 1861 strain, susceptible to antibiotics, and the lowest in the *E. faecalis* ATCC 51299 strain. The differences between the strains were not statistically significant (Table 2).

Table 2. The number of *Enterococcus* spp. recovered from air and the percentage reduction coefficient R [%].

Strain	The Average Number of Bacteria after Nebulization [CFU m^{-3}]	The Average Number of Bacteria after 20 min without RCI	Precipitate Factor $R_{withoutRCI}$ (K+) [%]	The Average Number of Bacteria after Using the Induct 750 [CFU m^{-3}]	Percentage of Reduction in the Number of Bacteria R_{RCI} [%]
Enterococcus faecalis PCM 1861	3.64×10^5 ($\pm 5.31 \times 10^4$) *	2.89×10^5 ($\pm 2.31 \times 10^4$)	20.60 ^{a}	8.72×10^2 ($\pm 7.05 \times 10^3$)	99.76 ^{b}
Enterococcus faecalis ATCC 51299	3.91×10^5 ($\pm 7.13 \times 10^4$) *	3.04×10^5 ($\pm 3.16 \times 10^4$)	22.25 ^{a}	3.89×10^4 ($\pm 7.05 \times 10^3$)	90.05 ^{b}
Enterococcus faecium ATCC 51559	3.18×10^5 ($\pm 8.23 \times 10^4$)	2.58×10^5 ($\pm 5.31 \times 10^4$)	18.99 ^{a}	1.25×10^3 ($\pm 9.63 \times 10^2$)	99.61 ^{b}

*—standard deviation. ^{a,b}—values marked with different letters differ statistically significant ($p \leq 0.05$).

3.3. Changes in the Number of *C. difficile* in the Air

The obtained results showed, similarly as in the case of *Enterococcus* spp., some fluctuations in the CFU number of tested bacilli present in the air after the suspension nebulization (Table 3). For this reason, it was decided to introduce an absolute reduction measure in the form of R [%].

After the nebulization, it was found that the CDI strain MXF-R/tox A/B/bin (+) most intensively formed bioaerosol, and the CDI PCR 027 strain—the worst (Table 3).

The use of RCI resulted in a decrease in the CFU number of all *C. difficile* strains tested in the air. The highest decrease, amounting to almost 95%, was found for the CDI MXF-R/tox A/B/bin(+) strain, and the lowest (over 64%) for the CDI PCR 027 strain (Table 3). The non-toxigenic CDI tox(−) strain was more resistant than the CDI MXF-R/tox A/B/bin(+) strain producing all toxins. Percentage reduction coefficients for the number of CDI tox(−) and CDI MXF-R/tox A/B/bin(+) strains were statistically significantly higher compared to the coefficient calculated for the CDI PCR 027 strain (Table 3).

Table 3. Number of *Clostridioides difficle* recovered from the air and the percentage reduction coefficient R [%].

Strain	The Average Number of Bacteria after Nebulization [CFU m^{-3}]	The Average Number of Bacteria after 20 min without RCI	Precipitate Factor $R_{withoutRCI}$ (K+) [%]	The Average Number of Bacteria after Using the Induct 750 [CFU m^{-3}]	Percentage of Reduction in the Number of Bacteria R_{RCI} [%]
CDI tox(−)	3.14×10^4 ($\pm 3.54 \times 10^2$) *	2.28×10^4 ($\pm 1.11 \times 10^2$)	27.36 ^{a}	5.15×10^3 ($\pm 7.21 \times 10^2$)	83.57 ^{b}
CDI MXF-R/ tox A/B/bin(+)	2.43×10^5 ($\pm 2.47 \times 10^4$)	1.74×10^5 ($\pm 2.26 \times 10^4$)	28.42 ^{a}	1.30×10^4 ($\pm 1.85 \times 10^3$)	94.65 ^{b}
CDI PCR 027	8.20×10^3 ($\pm 4.24 \times 10^2$)	6.03×10^4 ($\pm 3.81 \times 10^2$)	26.46 ^{a}	2.92×10^3 ($\pm 1.87 \times 10^2$)	64.45 ^{b}

CDI tox(−)—*C. difficile* non-toxinogenic strain; CDI MXF-R/tox A/B/bin(+)—*C. difficile* strain producing A, B and binary toxins and resistant to moxifloxacin; CDI PCR 027—*C. difficile* strain PCR-rybotype 027; *—standard deviation; ^{a,b}—values marked with different letters differ statistically significant ($p \leq 0.05$).

3.4. Changes in the Number of *Staphylococcus aureus* in the Air

Like in the case of species mentioned above, some fluctuations in the CFU number of tested *S. aureus* strains in the air after the suspensions nebulization were observed (Table 4). For this reason, it was decided to introduce an absolute reduction measure in the form of R [%].

The number of *S. aureus* reisolated from bioaerosol, after nebulization, range from 4.70 × 10^5 CFU m^{-3} for MRSA strain to 5.10 × 10^5 CFU m^{-3} for non-MRSA strain (Table 4).

The use of RCI resulted in a decrease in the CFU number of both *S. aureus* strains tested in the air. The greater number reduction (99.87%) was observed in case of non-MRSA strain. The statistically significant differences in R[%] were not shown among the tested strains (Table 4).

Table 4. The number of *Staphylococcus aureus* recovered from the air and the percentage reduction coefficient R [%].

Strain	The Average Number of Bacteria after Nebulization [CFU m^{-3}]	The Average Number of Bacteria after 20 min without RCI	Precipitate Factor $R_{withoutRCI}$ (K+) [%]	The Average Number of Bacteria after Using the Induct 750 [CFU m^{-3}]	Percentage of Reduction in the Number of Bacteria R_{RCI} [%]
Staphylococcus aureus MRSA	4.70 × 10^5 (±7.16 × 10^4) *	3.65 × 10^5 (±3.44 × 10^4)	22.34 ^{a}	2.06 × 10^4 (±1.72 × 10^4)	95.61 ^{b}
Staphylococcus aureus non-MRSA	5.10 × 10^5 (±1.12 × 10^5)	3.90 × 10^5 (±1.89 × 10^5)	23.60 ^{a}	6.50 × 10^2 (±9.22 × 10^1)	99.87 ^{b}

*—standard deviation; ^{a,b}—values marked with different letters differ statistically significant ($p \leq 0.05$).

4. Discussion

Microbiological air pollution in hospitals plays an important role in the spread of healthcare-associated infections [38–40]. Despite the methods of air purification used so far, e.g., ultraviolet germicidal irradiation (UVGI), HEPA filters, it is necessary to look for new, more effective technologies that enable the fight against increasingly virulent microbial strains that can spread through the aerogenic route. It is also important that new techniques are safe for people, because we spend over 90% of our time indoors and can be used while people are inside. RCI technology, unlike passive air purification methods, is an active method that purifies the air not only inside, but also outside the device. RCI has been shown to be an effective method for eliminating microbial contaminants, including viruses, vegetative forms, and persistent bacteria, from the surface [37,41–45]. It was found that this technology can be successfully used in many industries.

RCI method is quite a new approach to the indoor air disinfection issue. There are only very few publications in the available literature regarding the use of this method, and especially in relation to the experimental layout adopted in this research. Therefore, there are difficulties with regard to the results of own research to the work of other authors.

In the conducted experiment, the effectiveness of RCI against different strains of *Enterococcus* spp. and vegetative forms of *C. difiicile* were evaluated, paying attention to their virulence and resistance to antibiotics. The study showed the highest efficacy of RCI against *E. faecalis* PCM 1861 susceptible to antibiotics (R [%] = 99.76), but for all tested strains of *Enterococcus* spp., more than 90% efficiency in reducing the number of microorganisms in air after RCI has been demonstrated. In contrast, the lowest RCI efficacy was demonstrated for the *C. difficile* strain ribotype 027 (R [%] = 64.45). The use of RCI resulted in a decrease in the CFU number of both *S. aureus* strains tested in the air. The greater number reduction (99.87%) was observed in case of non-MRSA strain. Skowron et al. [37], higher efficacy of RCI against other spore forming bacteria, such as *Bacillus subtilis*, has been demonstrated (R [%] = 98.92). The lower susceptibility of *C. difficile* to RCI may be related to the virulence factors of these microorganisms, whereas this mechanism should be explained in subsequent studies. *C. difficile* rybotype 027 is an epidemic, high virulent strain that is characterized by more intense sporulation and production of large amounts of toxin A and B (16–23 times higher in vitro concentration than in case of other strains) [19,46–48]. The risk of aerogenic transfer of these microorganisms has been demonstrated by Roberts et al. [17], where the presence of these microorganisms in air samples collected in a hospital environment in Great Britain was demonstrated. Skowron et al. [37] showed the lowest RCI efficacy against *Clostridium sporogenes* spores (R [%] = 71.73). In other studies [44], we showed a reduction of *Klebsiella pneumoniae* NDM strains in the air at the level of 1.80 log CFU m^{-3} after using RCI technology. Skowron et al. [37] for *S. aureus* and *S. epidermidis* found a decrease in number amounted to 4–5 logarithmic units, and the percentage reduction rate was 99.9%. Also Grinshpun et al. [27] indicated that RCI technology caused a reduction of the *B. subtilis* spores in the 2.75 m^3 chamber. In the study, a chamber with a cubic capacity of 1.4 m^3 was used. The device manufacturer declares the device's efficiency to 70 m^3 (ActivTek, instruction of use Induct 750).

Skowron et al. [37] also demonstrated the differential efficacy of RCI on microorganisms in the air. The highest reduction coefficient (R [%] = 100) was demonstrated for *Escherichia coli* and *Candida albicans*. Effective elimination from the air was observed for *E. faecalis* ATCC 29212 (R [%] = 99.99), which, like *E. faecalis* PCM 1861, is sensitive to antibiotics [37]. Barabasz et al. [48] indicated that RCI was effective in rooms of cubature 20 and 45 m^3. The percentage reduction rate for the total number of *Staphylococcus* spp. and fungi ranged from 73.1% to 82.0% [42]. In turn, Wiktorczyk et al. [49] used the RCI module as a built-in element of the cabinet for storing endoscopes. The treatment influenced the meeting of microbiological criteria of air in the wardrobe [49].

In this study, the chamber nebulization time was 20 min, this is one of the parameters that can affect the effectiveness of eliminating pathogens from the air. In Skowron et al. study [37], the exposure time was also 20 min. However, in another study, we evaluated different exposure times [50] for the effectiveness of RCI technology. Skowron et al. [50], showed that the number of bacteria decreased with RCI exposure over time, which confirms previous studies. Skowron et al. [50] showed that the reduction of *S. aureus* from a stainless steel surface after 20 min exposure to RCI was 5.20 log CFU cm^{-2}. At the same time, Skowron et al. [50] found that *S. aureus* was the most resistant to RCI on the rubber surface. Grinshpun et al. [27] found that increasing the exposure time from 10 to 30 min increased the reduction in *B. subtilis* from 75 to 90%. Ortega et al. [34] showed that the 2 h RCI activity allowed a reduction of 90% of bacterial stainless steel plankton cells. The duration of RCI technology is crucial at the site of its application, especially in hospitals.

RCI technology based on reactions of photooxidation may in the near future become one of the most popular methods of air and surface cleaning, which is already in use in hospitals, museums, and schools [51]. Skorwon et al. [44] demonstrated the effectiveness of eliminating *K. pneumoniae* NDM from the materials used as hospital room equipment, including bedding. The effectiveness of this technology seems to be particularly important for highly virulent and antimicrobial resistant organisms that pose the greatest challenge for modern microbiology. In addition, Dimitrakopoulou et al. (2012), showed that the use of photocatalysis methods using UV-A/TiO_2 plays a role in the degradation of antibiotics present in the environment [52]. It is possible to use this technology in ventilation systems as support for existing solutions, e.g., HEPA filters, which will enable inactivation and removal of dead microorganisms from the air at the same time. RCI technology is mainly intended for cleaning inside the rooms and preventing the spread of microorganisms present in the hospital environment, e.g., between rooms, by personnel. RCI technology is based on photocatalysis. The emission of harmful substances has been proven, such as, ozone, aldehydes—formaldehyde and acetaldehyde, during photocatalysis, if this process occurs in an environment where a high concentration of volatile organic compounds (VOCs) is stated [30]. However, there is no research in the available literature on the production of such substances during the operation of RCI in rooms where there are people. A safe solution would be monitoring the concentrations of hazardous substances in places where RCI technology is used continuously when people are present in the room.

5. Conclusions

The obtained results indicate that the use of RCI may contribute to reducing the occurrence of dangerous pathogens (including MRSA) in the indoor air, and perhaps transmission and persistence in the environment. It is worth noticing that the RCI device should be taken into account in case of ventilation systems designing. However, in the future, more strains from different species should be examined. In addition, research is needed in real indoor environments.

Author Contributions: Conceptualization, K.S., K.G.-B., and S.K.; methodology, K.S., K.G.-B., and N.W.; validation, K.S. and N.W.; formal analysis, K.S. and K.J.S.; investigation, K.G.-B., S.K., and A.M.; resources, K.G.-B., S.K., and A.M.; writing—original draft preparation, N.W. and Z.B.; writing—review and editing, K.S., K.J.S., and Z.B.; visualization, N.W. and K.J.S.; supervision, K.S.; project administration, K.S. and E.G.-K.; funding acquisition, E.G.-K. All authors have read and agreed to the published version of the manuscript.

Funding: This research was financially supported by the Nicolaus Copernicus University with funds from the maintenance of the research potential of the Department of Microbiology PDB WF 536.

Conflicts of Interest: The authors declare no conflict of interest.

References

1. Beggs, C.; Knibbs, L.D.; Johnson, G.R.; Morawska, L. Environmental contamination and hospital-acquired infection: Factors that are easily overlooked. *Indoor Air* **2015**, *25*, 462–474. [CrossRef] [PubMed]
2. Jung, C.C.; Wu, P.C.; Tseng, C.H.; Su, H.J. Indoor air quality varies with ventilation types and working areas in hospitals. *Build. Environ.* **2015**, *85*, 190–195. [CrossRef]
3. Gilbert, Y.; Veillette, M.; Duchaine, C. Airborne bacteria and antibiotic resistance genes in hospital rooms. *Aerobiologia* **2010**, *26*, 185–194. [CrossRef]
4. Park, D.U.; Yeom, J.K.; Lee, W.J.; Lee, K.M. Assessment of the levels of airborne bacteria, gram-negative bacteria and fungi in hospital lobbies. *Int. J. Environ. Res. Publ. Health* **2013**, *10*, 541–555. [CrossRef] [PubMed]
5. Scaltriti, S.; Cencetti, S.; Rovesti, S.; Marchesi, I.; Bargellini, A.; Borella, P. Risk factors for particulate and microbial contamination of air in operating theatres. *J. Hosp. Infect.* **2007**, *66*, 320–326. [CrossRef]
6. Wan, G.H.; Chung, F.F.; Tang, C.S. Long-term surveillance of air quality in medical center operating rooms. *Am. J. Infect. Control* **2011**, *39*, 302–308. [CrossRef]
7. Shiomor, T.; Miyamoto, H.; Makishima, K.; Yoshida, M.; Fujiyoshi, T.; Udaka, T.; Inaba, T.; Hiraki, N. Evaluation of bedmaking-related airborne and surface methicillin-resistant *Staphylococcus aureus* contamination. *J. Hosp. Infect.* **2002**, *50*, 30–35. [CrossRef]
8. Atkinson, J.; Chartier, Y.; Pessoa-Silva, C.L.; Jensen, P.; Li, Y.; Seto, W.H. *Natural Ventilation for Infection Control in Health-Care Settings*; World Health Organization: Geneva, Switzerland, 2009. Available online: https://www.ncbi.nlm.nih.gov/books/NBK143277/ (accessed on 8 April 2020).
9. Lim, T.; Chob, J.; Kim, B.S. The predictions of infection risk of indoor airborne transmission of diseases in high-rise hospitals: Tracer gas simulation. *Energy Build.* **2010**, *42*, 1172–1181. [CrossRef]
10. Wallner, P.; Munoz, U.; Tappler, P.; Wanka, A.; Kundi, M.; Shelton, J.F.; Hutter, H.P. Indoor environmental quality in mechanically ventilated, energy-efficient buildings vs. conventional buildings. *Int. J. Environ. Res. Public Health* **2015**, *12*, 14132–14147. [CrossRef]
11. Gao, M.; An, T.; Li, G.; Nie, X.; Yip, H.L.; Zhao, H.; Wong, P.K. Genetic studies of the role of fatty acid and coenzyme A in photocatalytic inactivation of *Escherichia coli*. *Water Res.* **2012**, *46*, 3951–3957. [CrossRef]
12. Hayden, M.K. Insights into the epidemiology and control of infection with vancomycin-resistant enterococci. *Clin. Infect. Dis.* **2000**, *31*, 1058–1065. [CrossRef] [PubMed]
13. Rathnayake, I.U.; Hargreaves, M.; Huygens, F. Antibiotic resistance and virulence traits in clinical and environmental *Enterococcus faecalis* and *Enterococcus faecium* isolates. *Syst. Appl. Microbiol.* **2012**, *35*, 326–333. [CrossRef] [PubMed]
14. Collins, J.; Auchtung, J.M. Control of *Clostridium difficile* infection by defined microbial communities. *Microbiol. Spectr.* **2017**, *5*, 1–25.
15. Awad, M.M.; Johanesen, P.A.; Carter, G.P.; Rose, E.; Lyras, D. *Clostridium difficile* virulence factors: Insights into an anaerobic spore-forming pathogen. *Gut Microbes* **2014**, *5*, 579–593. [CrossRef] [PubMed]
16. Quesada-Gómez, C.; López-Ureña, D.; Acuña-Amador, L.; Villalobos-Zúñiga, M.; Du, T.; Freire, R.; Guzmán-Verri, C.; del Mar Gamboa-Coronado, M.; Lawley, T.D.; Moreno, E.; et al. Emergence of an outbreak-associated *Clostridium difficile* variant with increased virulence. *J. Clin. Microbiol.* **2015**, *53*, 1216–1226. [CrossRef] [PubMed]
17. Roberts, K.; Smith, C.F.; Snelling, A.M.; Kerr, K.G.; Banfield, K.R.; Sleigh, P.A.; Beggs, C.B. Aerial dissemination of *Clostridium difficile* spores. *BMC Infect. Dis.* **2008**, *8*, 1–6. [CrossRef]

18. Best, E.L.; Fawley, W.N.; Parnell, P.; Wilcox, M.H. The potential for airborne dispersal of *Clostridium difficile* from symptomatic patients. *Clin. Infect. Dis.* **2010**, *50*, 1450–1457. [CrossRef]
19. Carlson, P.E.; Kaiser, A.M.; McColm, S.A.; Bauer, J.M.; Young, V.B.; Aronoff, D.M.; Hanna, P.C. Variation in germination of *Clostridium difficile* clinical isolates correlates to disease severity. *Anaerobe* **2015**, *33*, 64–70. [CrossRef]
20. Gerding, D.N.; Muto, C.A.; Owens, R.C. Measures to control and prevent *Clostridium difficile* infection. *Clin. Infect. Dis.* **2008**, *46*, S43–S49. [CrossRef]
21. Fawley, W.N.; Parnell, P.; Verity, P.; Freeman, J.; Wilcox, M.H. Molecular epidemiology of endemic *Clostridium difficile* infection and the significance of subtypes of the United Kingdom epidemic strain (PCR ribotype 1). *J. Clin. Microbiol.* **2005**, *43*, 2685–2696. [CrossRef]
22. Snelling, A.M.; Beggs, C.B.; Kerr, K.G.; Shepherd, S.J. Spores of *Clostridium difficile* in Hospital Air. *Clin. Infect. Dis.* **2010**, *51*, 1104–1105. [CrossRef] [PubMed]
23. Aires de Sousa, M.; Lencastre, H. Bridges from hospitals to the laboratory: Genetic portraits of methicillin-resistant *Staphylococcus aureus* clones. *Pathog. Dis.* **2004**, *40*, 101–111.
24. Berning, C.; Lanckohr, C.; Baumgartner, H.; Drescher, M.; Becker, K.; Peters, G.; Köck, R.; Kahl, B.C. Fatal infections caused by methicillin-resistant *Staphylococcus aureus* of clonal complex 398: Case presentations and molecular epidemiology. *JMM Case Rep.* **2015**, *2*, e000024. [CrossRef]
25. Shirmori, T.; Miyamoto, H.; Makishima, K. Significance of airbone transmission of methicillin-resistant *Staphylococus aureus* in an otolaryngology-head and neck surgery unit. *Arch. Otolaryngol. Head Neck Surg.* **2001**, *127*, 644–648. [CrossRef] [PubMed]
26. Space Fundation, Radiant Catalytic Ionization Air & Water Purification. Available online: http://www.spacefoundation.org/programs/space-certification/certified-products/space-technology/radiant-catalytic-ionization-air (accessed on 10 February 2020).
27. Grinshpun, S.A.; Adhikari, A.; Honda, T.; Kim, K.Y.; Toivola, M.; Rao, K.S. Reponen, Control of aerosol contaminants in indoor air: Combining the particle concentration reduction with microbial inactivation. *Environ. Sci. Technol.* **2007**, *41*, 606–612. [CrossRef] [PubMed]
28. Binas, V.; Venieri, D.; Kotzias, D.; Kiriakidis, G. Modified TiO_2 based photocatalysts for improved air and health quality. *J. Materiomics* **2017**, *3*, 3–16. [CrossRef]
29. Gao, W.; Howden, B.P.; Stinear, T.P. Evolution of virulence in *Enterococcus faecium*, a hospital-adapted opportunistic pathogen. *Curr. Opin. Microbiol.* **2017**, *41*, 76–82. [CrossRef]
30. Hodgson, A.I.; Destaillats, H.; Sullivan, D.P.; Fisk, W.J. Performance of ultraviolet photocatalytic oxidation for indoor air cleaning applications. *Indoor Air* **2007**, *17*, 305–316. [CrossRef]
31. Mo, J.; Zhang, Y.; Xu, Q.; Lamson, J.J.; Zhao, R. Photocatalytic purification of volatile organic compounds in indoor air: A literature review. *Atmos. Environ.* **2009**, *43*, 2229–2246. [CrossRef]
32. Huang, G.; Xia, D.; An, T.; Ng, T.W.; Yip, H.Y.; Li, G.; Zhao, H.; Wong, P.K. Dual roles of capsular extracellular polymeric substances in photocatalytic inactivation of *Escherichia coli*: Comparison of *E. coli* BW25113 and isogenic mutants. *Appl. Environ. Microbiol.* **2015**, *81*, 5174–5183. [CrossRef]
33. Yang, X.; Wang, Y. Photocatalytic effect on plasmid DNA damage under different UV irradiation time. *Build. Environ.* **2008**, *43*, 253–257. [CrossRef]
34. Ortega, M.T.; Franken, L.J.; Hatesohl, P.R.; Marsden, L.J. Efficacy of ecoquest radiant catalytic Ionization cell and breeze at ozone generator at reducing microbial populations on stainless steel surfaces. *J. Rapid Meth. Aut. Mic.* **2007**, *5*, 359–368. [CrossRef]
35. ActivTek. Instruction of Use Induct 750 Product. Available online: http://activtek.pl/wp-content/uploads/2014/12/INDUCT-750-Spec-Sheet.pdf (accessed on 10 February 2020).
36. WHO. *Air Quality Guidelines for Particulate Matter, Ozone, Nitrogen Dioxide and Sulfur Dioxide Global Update 2005 Summary of Risk Assessment*; World Health Organization: Geneva, Switzerland, 2005.
37. Skowron, K.; Grudlewska, K.; Kwiecińska-Piróg, J.; Gryń, G.; Śrutek, M.; Gospodarek-Komkowska, E. Efficacy of radiant catalytic ionization to reduce bacterial populations in air and on different surfaces. *Sci. Total Environ.* **2018**, *610–611*, 111–120. [CrossRef] [PubMed]
38. Zhang, Y.H.; Leung, N.H.; Cowling, B.J.; Yang, Z.F. Role of viral bioaerosols in nosocomial infections and measures for prevention and control. *J. Aerosol Sci.* **2018**, *117*, 200–211.

39. Fletcher, L.A.; Noakes, C.J.; Beggs, C.B.; Sleigh, P.A. The importance of bioaerosols in hospital infections and the potential for control using germicidal ultraviolet irradiation. In Proceedings of the 1st Seminar on Applied Aerobiology, Murcia, Spain, 20 May 2004.
40. Lai, K.; Nasir, Z.A.; Taylor, J. Bioaerosols and hospital infections. *Aerosol Sci.* **2014**, *117*, 271–289.
41. Matsunaga, T.; Tamoda, R.; Nakajima, T.; Wake, H. Photoelectrochemical sterilization of microbial cells by semiconductor powers. *FEMS Microbiol. Lett.* **1985**, *29*, 211–214. [CrossRef]
42. Gogniat, G.; Thyssen, M.; Denis, M.; Pulgarin, C.; Dukan, S. The bactericidal effect of TiO_2 photocatalysis in volves adsorption on to catalyst and the loss of membrane integrity. *FEMS Microbiol. Lett.* **2006**, *258*, 18–24. [CrossRef]
43. Paspaltsis, I.; Kotta, K.; Lagoudaki, R.; Grigoriadis, N.; Poulios, I.; Sklaviadis, T. Titanium dioxide photocatalytic inactivation of prions. *J. Gen. Virol.* **2006**, *87*, 3125–3130. [CrossRef]
44. Skowron, K.; Wiktorczyk, N.; Kwiecińska-Piróg, J.; Sękowska, A.; Wałecka-Zacharska, E.; Gospodarek-Komkowska, E. Elimination of *Klebsiella pneumoniae* NDM from the air and selected surfaces in hospital using radiant catalytic ionization. *Lett. Appl. Microbiol.* **2019**, *69*, 333–338. [CrossRef]
45. McDonald, L.C.; Killgore, G.E.; Thompson, A.; Owens, R.C.; Kazakova, S.V.; Sambol, S.P.; Johnson, S.; Gerding, D.N. An epidemic, toxin gene-variant strain of *Clostridium difficile*. *N. Engl. J. Med.* **2005**, *353*, 2433–2441. [CrossRef]
46. Smits, W.K.; Lyras, D.; Lacy, D.B.; Wilcox, M.H.; Kuijper, E.J. *Clostridium difficile* infection. *Nat. Rev. Dis. Primers* **2012**, *2*, 16–20. [CrossRef] [PubMed]
47. Warny, M.; Pepin, J.; Fang, A.; Killgore, G.; Thompson, A.; Brazier, J.; Frost, E.; McDonald, L.C. Toxin production by an emerging strain of *Clostridium difficile* associated with outbreaks of severe disease in North America and Europe. *Lancet* **2005**, *36*, 1079–1084. [CrossRef]
48. Barabasz, W. The Results of the Research Carried out in University of Agriculture in Krakow about Efficacy of RCI Technology. 2014. Available online: http://activtek.pl/wp-content/uploads/2014/07/Uniwersytet-Rolniczy.pdf (accessed on 10 February 2020).
49. Wiktorczyk, N.; Kwiecińska-Piróg, J.; Skowron, K.; Michalska, A.; Zalas-Więcek, P.; Białucha, A.; Budzyńska, A.; Grudlewska-Buda, K.; Prażyńska, M.; Gospodarek-Komkowska, E. Assessment of endoscope cleaning and disinfection efficacy, and the impact of endoscope storage on the microbiological safety level. *J. App. Microb.* **2019**, *128*, 1503–1513. [CrossRef] [PubMed]
50. Skowron, K.; Wałecka-Zacharska, E.; Grudlewska, K.; Kwiecińska-Piróg, J.; Wiktorczyk, N.; Kowalska, M.; Paluszak, Z.; Kosek-Paszkowska, K.; Brożek, K.; Korkus, J.; et al. Effect of selected environmental factors on the microbicidal effectiveness of radiant catalytic ionization. *Front. Microbiol.* **2020**, *10*. [CrossRef] [PubMed]
51. ActivTek. Documents About Use of Product. Available online: http://activtek.pl/dokumenty/ (accessed on 10 February 2020).
52. Dimitrakopoulou, D.; Rethemiotaki, I.; Frontistis, Z.; Xekoukoulotakis, N.P.; Venieri, D.; Mantzavinos, D. Degradation, mineralization and antibiotic inactivation of amoxicillin by UV-A/TiO_2 photocatalysis. *J. Environ. Manag.* **2012**, *98*, 168–174. [CrossRef] [PubMed]

MDPI
St. Alban-Anlage 66
4052 Basel
Switzerland
Tel. +41 61 683 77 34
Fax +41 61 302 89 18
www.mdpi.com

Atmosphere Editorial Office
E-mail: atmosphere@mdpi.com
www.mdpi.com/journal/atmosphere

www.ingramcontent.com/pod-product-compliance
Lightning Source LLC
LaVergne TN
LVHW070541100526
838202LV00012B/344
* 9 7 8 3 0 3 6 5 2 2 6 4 7 *